Advance Praise for
Beyond the Stethoscope

"Dr. Janette is an angel on Earth—she has more medical knowledge and compassion than anyone I've ever met. In her new book, *Beyond the Stethoscope: Miracles in Medicine*, you will get to meet this remarkable woman who reminds me every day to be gracious under pressure, and you'll be convinced that miracles happen right in front of your eyes."

–Dana Perino, *America's Newsroom*

"Dr. Janette Nesheiwat's *Beyond the Stethoscope* offers a raw and captivating glimpse into the world of a true medical warrior. From battling the front lines of Covid to navigating the aftermath of natural disasters and global conflicts, her journey is a testament to grit, compassion, and unwavering dedication. Through her experiences, Dr. Nesheiwat reminds us that true miracles in medicine are forged by the relentless commitment of those who strive to make a difference."

–Congressman Mike Waltz, US Army Green Beret, Colonel

"A must read! I'm inspired by Dr. Nesheiwat's dedication to serving others in the name of Jesus Christ. Her extraordinary service is documented in *Beyond the Stethoscope: Miracles in Medicine* where she showcases the power of Jesus guiding her work leading challenging and dangerous medical missions throughout the world. This book is a reminder of the blessings that unfold when we trust in God's love."

–Ainsley Earhardt, Co-host *Fox & Friends*

"A truly remarkable read. I cried, smiled, was outraged, and couldn't put it down."

–Hayat Zeidan, RN

"As a doctor myself, I found the journey of Dr. Janette deeply moving and profoundly relatable. With raw honesty and poignant insight, she captures the essence of doctors' lives and the convoluted relationships with patients. The joy, sorrows, and triumphs—she talks about it all—making her book a great read for anyone."

–Dr. Sammy Turner

BEYOND THE STETHOSCOPE

MIRACLES IN MEDICINE

DR. JANETTE NESHEIWAT

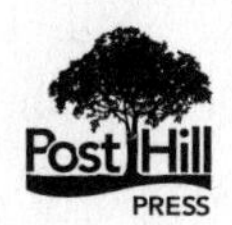

A POST HILL PRESS BOOK
ISBN: 979-8-88845-651-4
ISBN (eBook): 979-8-88845-652-1

Beyond the Stethoscope:
Miracles in Medicine

Cover design by Jim Villaflores
Cover photo by Fadil Berisha

Proceeds will be donated to CHARM, the Children Are Magical Foundation.
ChildrenAreMagical.org

All people, locations, events, and situations are portrayed to the best of the author's memory. While all of the events described are true, many names and identifying details have been changed to protect the privacy of the people involved. Descriptions of medical treatments and diagnoses are purely for illustrative purposes, and are not meant to constitute medical advice. In all instances, readers should consult with their own medical professional.

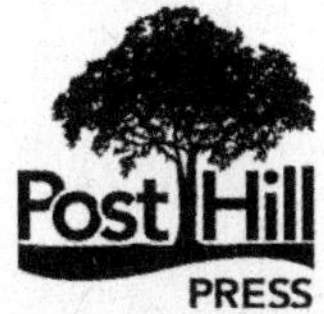

Post Hill Press
New York • Nashville
posthillpress.com

Published in the United States of America
1 2 3 4 5 6 7 8 9 10

To my beautiful mom and the world's greatest nurse,
Hayat Nesheiwat, RN, and all my brothers and
sisters for all your love and encouragement.

TABLE OF CONTENTS

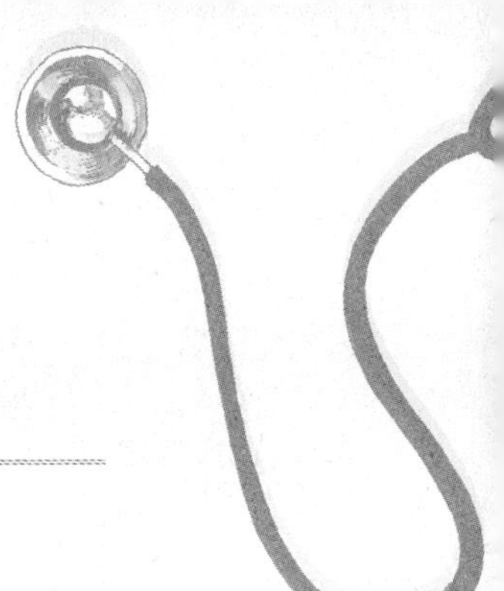

PREFACE

> The point is art never stopped a war and never got anybody a job. That was never its function. Art cannot change events. But it can change people. It can affect people so that they are changed...because people are changed by art—enriched, ennobled, encouraged—they then act in a way that may affect the course of events.
>
> —Leonard Bernstein, iconic American composer and conductor, in the documentary film *Bernstein's Wall*

The same can be said of the healing arts.

Healthcare professionals do not control the outcomes, although some may think they do. We are the hands of God on Earth. We are His relay. Healing arts create the opportunity to affect the course of events.

There will always be natural and man-made catastrophes. Many generations continue to live through multiple infectious outbreaks, fires, earthquakes, floods, and we are not done. This is our hero's journey, persevering and passing down our actionable faith.

> "You are the light of the world. A city set on a hill cannot be hidden; nor does anyone light a lamp and put it under a bas-

> ket, but on the lampstand, and it gives
> light to all who are in the house.
> "Let your light shine before men in
> such a way that they may see your good
> works, and glorify your Father who is in
> heaven" (Matthew 5:14–16 NKJV).

These are my stories to educate *Beyond the Stethoscope* and demonstrate the testimony of everyday miracles.

In hope and healing,
Janette

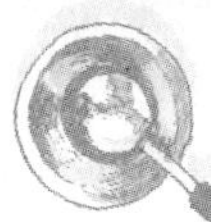

INTRODUCTION

When I was thirteen years old, I helplessly watched my dear father dying from an accident as blood was spurting everywhere. It was the most traumatic sight that turned my life upside down. It's an image that killed my insides for many years, and as I got older, it became difficult for me to recover. I couldn't save his life. I was in such shock. I was helpless and so useless. The trauma of that moment clung to me like a relentless shadow, unraveling the fabric of my young life and leaving me in a perpetual state of devastation. Over the years, my mother and siblings helped me tremendously to cope with this trauma. It was their support, encouragement, and my mother's inspirational guidance to have me look at life in another perspective by helping others, by caring for the less fortunate, by sharing, and learning to save lives. This was the start of my personal journey in life to become a physician and enter the world of healing arts to help me cope with the pain of the past and find a way to make up for one lost life. So, I was on my own healing process to save as many lives as I could with God's help. This calling led me to the front lines of humanity's most perilous moments. This is how my story begins and why I was driven to help so many at every hazardous, dangerous, life-threatening disaster area: hurricanes, earthquakes, floods, tsunamis, war zones, and the epicenter of COVID in New York City where I treated over twenty thousand COVID-related patients.

I am the daughter of immigrant parents who came to America searching for the American Dream. I am no different than the millions of others who also immigrated to America to find their dream, only mine had some nightmares, miracles, even some near-death experiences. I was born in New York but grew up in a small town one hour north of Orlando. My parents moved our large family to Florida where they loved the agriculture, and the weather was summer all year round. I studied at the University of South Florida where I enrolled in an Army ROTC program. I did basic training in Fort Lewis, Washington, and completed my medical training at the University of Arkansas where I served as chief resident. My goal fulfilled, I became a board-certified physician and moved back to New York where I worked at a healthcare center on 42nd Street in Times Square that was a battlefront war zone region like an ER. It was nonstop walk-ins, never knowing what was coming in the front door. It was a continuous surge of unpredictability. In an average week, I saw a multitude of cases from crushed bones, skulls, and lacerations to heart attacks, strokes, appendicitis, stabbings, gang-related gunshot wounds, prostitutes, rapes, and more. It was never a dull day or night. I was well acquainted with the trauma and desperation that lingered from treating hundreds of injured patients from Hurricane Katrina in 2005, working with bare hands in Haiti after the deadly 2010 earthquake, and witnessing the tragedies in Joplin, Missouri, after its horrific 2011 tornado that ravaged the town to caring for refugees fleeing the bombing and the destruction of their homes in the war zone of Ukraine. I really was baptized by fire! But I, as well as my country, our governments, hospitals, and the American healthcare system, was not ready for the disaster and the fear that was about to hit our country, our civilization, as it did with the coming pandemic.

RAGE, FEAR, ANGER

As a doctor, I was worried when COVID hit back in 2019/2020. I will never forget the first telecast of Italy locked down with hundreds dying; it was shocking. It all felt surreal, like we were living through a biblical plague. I witnessed the ravages of the virus firsthand at the hospital, and my heart ached for all those suffering. The weight of their pain and fear hung heavy on my shoulders. I cried out silently for strength, remembering Isaiah 41:10 KJV, "So do not fear, for I am with you; do not be dismayed, for I am your God. I will strengthen you and help you; I will uphold you with my righteous right hand."

But as time passed, the fear turned into something more insidious—anger and rage: anger at the virus for taking lives so ruthlessly, anger at the misinformation spreading like wildfire, and rage at the politicians who seemed more interested in their own agendas than in saving lives. The anger boiled within me, and I recalled the words of Ephesians 4:26 KJV, "In your anger do not sin: Do not let the sun go down while you are still angry." But it seemed impossible not to be furious in the face of such suffering.

GREAT DECEPTION

There was indeed a lot of deception. Initially, people didn't take it seriously. China was deceptive, and our government administration was unprepared for this pandemic. As a doctor, I felt the weight of this deception in ways I could never have imagined. Every day, I saw the real and devastating consequences of the deception and misinformation that had swirled around this virus. I was wary of many people. Even Matthew 7:15 KJV tells us, "Beware of false prophets, who come to you in sheep's clothing but inwardly are ravenous wolves." This verse was a stark reminder of the deception we faced from China and even within our society.

I couldn't help but think about how deception had played a significant role in spreading the virus. The misinformation, the conflicting reports, and the hidden truths contributed to the chaos. More often during those days, I found myself questioning the very core of our society's values and ethics.

HEAL THYSELF

I feel I have come a long way from growing up in a small town, traveling the world, and having the privilege of becoming a doctor of the healing arts. I consider these to be blessings that God has bestowed on me for being able to impact people and save many lives.

WHO ARE YOU HOLDING IN YOUR DUNGEON?

I have come to realize God plans for me, and whatever path He has chosen for me, I wonder what more my future holds. Ever since witnessing my father's death at a young age, I have felt a profound sense of duty to heal, but it came with an emotional toll that I hadn't anticipated.

I've come to understand that healing others is a noble calling, but it's equally important to heal oneself. It's like the words in Matthew 7:5 NIV, "You hypocrite, first take the plank out of your eye, and then you will see clearly to remove the speck from your brother's eye." To truly help others, I must first heal my wounds and tend to my spiritual well-being.

MORALITY

I have seen so much tragedy, so much devastation, so much of man's inhumanity to humanity. I am often left numb, and yet I am genuinely thankful to God for each day he allows me to live and give and not take anything for granted.

The weight of suffering and loss can be overwhelming, but 2 Corinthians 1:3–4 NIV reminds me of my purpose: "Praise be to the God and Father of our Lord Jesus Christ, the Father of compassion and the God of all comfort, who comforts us in all our troubles so that we can comfort those in any trouble with the comfort we receive from God." I draw strength from this promise, knowing that my healing journey is intertwined with the healing of others.

DO NO HARM

Indeed, all my life, I have lived by the mantra "do no harm." I am saddened beyond words due to the pain and suffering that surrounds us each day. Needless violence, abuse, mental illness—these are the burdens I confront as a doctor. It is not just a profession; it is a sacred calling, a mission to heal, comfort, and bring solace to those who endure the harshest trials of existence.

The concept of "do no harm" is not just a mantra; it's a solemn vow, a sacred promise. But as a healer, I am not exempt from the wounds of this world since I bear the scars of witnessing lives cut short and the trauma on their faces when they are in the darkest days of their lives. The weight of these emotions can sometimes be overwhelming, but I am reminded of Galatians 6:9 NIV, "Let us not become weary in doing good, for at the proper time we will reap a harvest if we do not give up." I must persevere, for amid despair, healing is possible, and I must be the vessel through which it flows.

FALSE ASSUMPTIONS

Not everyone who smiles with you is a friend. Not everyone you talk to is supportive or understands. Life is hard, people are struggling, and you don't know what it's like to be in someone else's shoes, let alone their life. The recent death of one of my dear colleagues still shocks me. We worked together during our medical residency. A nice father of four, he committed suicide, and I can't fathom why. There was no hint of the darkness that must have been lurking beneath his jovial exterior.

Amid this tragedy, I couldn't help but reflect on the false assumptions we often make about people. We assume that a smile means happiness, that success equates to inner peace, and that our colleagues are coping just as well as we are. It's a sobering reminder of the complexities of human nature and the hidden struggles that many endure.

Proverbs 14:10 NIV comes to mind: "Each heart knows its bitterness, and no one else can share its joy." It reminds me that we can never truly understand the depths of someone else's pain.

HOPE FOR TODAY AND THE FUTURE

I live on hope and optimism for a better day ahead always. My strong faith in God and how He will always provide and see us through is imprinted in my heart and mind.

They say hospital walls have witnessed more prayers than church walls. I can affirm this as a doctor: the hospital walls have seen the darkest moments of human suffering and absorbed the tears and prayers of countless souls. But I find the strength to go on there, in this crucible of pain and healing.

As I walk through the hospital corridors, I see patients and their families clinging to hope, just as I do. In these moments, I'm reminded of Romans 12:12 NIV: "Be joyful in hope, patient in affliction, faithful in prayer." The weight of our profession is immense, but so is the power of hope—hope for today, tomorrow, and the future.

STRUGGLE, PAIN, SUFFERING, ADVERSITY

It felt like I was wading through an endless storm, a tempest of emotions and raw trauma that threatened to engulf me—every day brought new challenges, new doubts, and new fears. I was a doctor, a healer of others, but I found myself desperately trying to heal the unhealable, at times feeling like I couldn't do enough to ease their pain. And in those quiet moments, I'd apologize to myself for not being stronger or having all the answers.

Confusion was a constant companion; I was lost in the maze of my thoughts, perplexed by the complexity of human suffering. On such days, I would turn to my Bible for solace and guidance. I have come to accept that these struggles will always be a part of life, but I will prevail with faith as my anchor; 2 Corinthians 4:8–9 NIV resonates with me: "We are hard pressed on every side, but not crushed; perplexed, but not in despair; persecuted, but not abandoned; struck down, but not destroyed."

SAFELY TRUST GOD

The difficulties of this life are opportunities to walk closely with our Savior and know Him better. In the book of Psalms, David was weighed down with many woes and worries, and we all can undoubtedly identify with his desire to "fly away and be at rest."

Casting your cares upon God means releasing them fully into His control and allowing Him to be your "place of refuge from the stormy wind and heavy gale" (Psalm 55:8 NASB). Still, I struggled with this concept for a long time. I questioned why God would allow so much suffering and why He would place these burdens upon us. And then, I started praying consistently and fervently. I was feeling overwhelmed with the pain, but I put all my trust in the Lord: "Trust in the Lord with all your heart and lean not on your own understanding; in all your ways submit to him, and he will make your paths straight" (Proverbs 3:5–6 NIV).

I realized that my role was not just about medical expertise but also about faith and trust—I had to trust that God would guide me through the darkest times and that He would provide the strength to heal my patients and me.

In health,
Dr. Janette

SPLIT-SECOND LIFESAVING DECISIONS—DOCTOR'S INTUITION

In the heart-stopping, adrenaline-fueled world of emergency medicine, it's an everyday occurrence to fight for the life of an unfamiliar face, a patient in the ER. Yet, when that face is one you've known since childhood, the stakes feel infinitely higher.

I was visiting my cousin, who was relaxing watching TV but told me she had belly pain. I pressed on her belly; it was mildly sore. Yet, something inside me stirred. I postponed my 4 p.m. flight to 7 p.m., deciding to stay a little longer and observe her closely for an hour or so, like a silent sentinel watching for signs of trouble, just to be sure.

As the minutes ticked by, her pain escalated. I decided we were going to the ER. Perhaps it was appendicitis, I reasoned. But as she struggled to dress, her strength failed her, and she crumpled to the floor, unconscious. My heart pounded as I dialed 911, trying to rouse her while waiting for the ambulance.

ECHOES IN THE HALLWAY

The paramedics arrived swiftly, administering an IV and transferring her onto a stretcher. We rushed off to the ER, where we were left waiting in the hallway. As I watched her, her eyes rolled back, her skin turned a frightening shade of blue, and she lost consciousness again. Panic gripped me. I called out for help once, twice, but no one came. The third time, driven by a primal need to save her life at any cost, desperation fueled my shout: "I need F*****G help over here NOW!"

My plea finally caught someone's attention but not without consequence. Security escorted me out of the ER, blind to the dire situation unfolding before their eyes. I hadn't revealed my medical background; sometimes, it can create unnecessary tension. But I knew the severity of her condition, and I feared for her life. If I hadn't pushed them, if I hadn't fought for her, she would not have made it. She was on the brink of death.

DOCTOR'S RACE AGAINST TIME

The diagnosis was grim—a ruptured ectopic pregnancy had caused her to hemorrhage internally. The surgeon was tied up in another operation, and my cousin was slipping in and out of consciousness, unable to answer their questions. I stepped in, providing the vital information they needed. They rushed her into the operating room, starting a blood transfusion as she had already lost around three liters of blood—a blood loss that's not usually compatible with life.

As I paced the hospital corridor, sleepless and weary, I felt a profound sense of gratitude. I was there, at the right place and at the right time, to save her life. It was a night that etched itself in my memory, a stark reminder of the fragility of life and the strength of family bonds. The experience drained me yet filled me with a newfound appreciation for my profession and the miracles it could perform.

It was as if divine intervention had played a part, guiding my actions and keeping both of us alive. I remembered Philippians 4:6 NIV—even when worries overcome us, this verse reminds us that we still have hope. It comforts and emphasizes the importance of "prayer and petition" and thanksgiving as the spirit through which we approach God.

Fear is a natural response to being diagnosed with sickness or watching a loved one battle sickness. Even in the most trying times, trust your instincts and never underestimate the power of persistence and love. When we act with genuine concern and determination, even amid overwhelming odds, we can be the beacon of hope that guides others through their darkest hours.

Sometimes, destiny puts us in places not just for our journey but to be a critical chapter in someone else's story. In the tapestry of life, some threads are destined to cross at just the right moment, and such was the day for me and my cousin.

I WILL NEVER FORGET, BRENDA

This is the story about my patient, Brenda, who accidentally drove her motorcycle off a mountain cliff in Arkansas. Knowing that it was a serious, potentially life-threatening injury, a helicopter was enroute. When the ambulance got to the bottom of the cliff, they saw she was alive, so they canceled the helicopter midflight.

One hour later, Brenda was brought to the ER where I was working in a rural three-bed ER in Eureka Springs. I was stunned that she suddenly came through the doors because I knew this was a serious trauma. We immediately put IVs in her, and I called a helicopter to transport her out of state to Missouri, which is the nearest trauma center. Time was ticking! It was the golden hour, that critical time after a traumatic injury when medical treatment is most effective, and chances of survival are best. I knew she had internal bleeding. The helicopter picked her up from my ER, and by the time it landed in Springfield, she coded, went unconscious, and CPR was performed. They rushed her straight into the operating room after a focused assessment with sonography in trauma (FAST) ultrasound. There was a high chance she was going to bleed to death that night. I got down on my hands and knees and prayed in the doctors' lounge. "Please God, keep her alive; please God, let her live," I remember praying so hard.

I called the hospital to check on her. They said she was still in the operating room. She had broken ribs, collapsed lungs, and bleeding into her chest and abdomen. I called again a few hours later. They said she was still in the operating room.

I fell asleep in the doctors' lounge at four in the morning.

The third time I called, I asked what room she was in because I thought if they gave me a room number, I would know she had not died. I was praying for a room number.

The nurse put her hand over the phone—I tried to make out what was being said. She was asking the patient for permission to talk to me. I heard in the background the patient saying, "Tell the doctor I said thank you." I broke down in tears because I knew she was a miracle in medicine. I'll never forget her. God kept her alive.

POWER OF PRAYER

I strongly believe in the power of prayer—in early 2023, during a Monday Night Football game between the Buffalo Bills and the Cincinnati Bengals, Bills Safety Damar Hamlin collided with the Bengals wide receiver Tee Higgins, Damar then collapsed and became unresponsive. CPR was started.

At one point in time the entire nation was united in praying for Damar as we all witnessed his collapse on the field after he was struck in the chest and suffered from commotio cordis, a heart condition causing his heart to stop beating properly.

I remember I was on air with Lawrence Jones talking about Damar's critical condition. I nearly said to Lawrence, live on air, let's bow our heads and close our eyes and pray for him right now. Damar's recovery was a testament to the power of prayer and the strength of faith.

Damar later said "Sudden cardiac arrest is something I never would have chosen to be a part of my story, but that's because our own visions are too small even when we think we see the whole picture. My vision was about playing in the NFL and being the best player I could be, but God's plan was to have a purpose greater than any game in this world."

People from all walks of life unified to lift him in prayer, highlighting the profound impact of God's blessings, his purpose for each of us and the importance of prayer in times of both crisis and recovery.

Just as it was with my experience praying for my patient Brenda and also joining with the nation to pray for Damar, the power of prayer is not to be underestimated. We are reminded of this in Matthew 21:22 NIV "If you believe, you will receive whatever you ask for in prayer."

THE MIRACLE OF DIVINE PROTECTION: GOD'S SHIELD OVER PRESIDENT DONALD TRUMP

In the realm of medicine, we often witness extraordinary moments that defy logic, science, and human understanding. These instances remind us of the presence of a higher power orchestrating the events of our lives. One such remarkable event is the divine protection of President Donald Trump, a moment that transcended the ordinary and showcased the miraculous intervention of God's hand.

July 13, 2024 was a day like any other, with the usual hustle and bustle of activities surrounding President Trump as he headed to Pennsylvania for a rally. The air was charged with anticipation as he prepared to address a large gathering of supporters. Unbeknownst to many, that day would be marked by a miraculous event that would leave an indelible mark on the hearts of those who witnessed it.

As the crowd gathered, the atmosphere was electric with excitement and fervor. However, hidden in the shadows of a rooftop was an individual with malicious intent, armed with a weapon and a heart filled with ill will. The assailant's plan was clear—to bring harm to President Trump, to end his life with a single, fatal shot.

The United States Secret Service is renowned for its meticulous planning and unwavering dedication to protecting the nation's leaders. The Secret Service operates with a multifaceted approach to security, incorporating physical protection, intelligence gathering, and advance planning. Before any event, the Secret Service conducts thorough site surveys, identifying potential threats and securing the perimeter. Agents work closely with local law enforcement and event organizers to ensure every aspect of the venue is secure. Medical teams are always on standby to provide immediate care if necessary. But nothing is 100 percent in life.

As the event commenced, the crowd's cheers filled the air, creating a cacophony of sound. In the midst of this, a moment of stillness descended—a moment that felt like time itself had paused. The assailant who witnesses saw climb a rooftop, took aim, his finger on the trigger, ready to unleash his deadly intent. But as he pulled the trigger, the bullet exited the chamber, something miraculous happened. Trump turned his head a mere inch such that the bullet missed his brain and only grazed his ear. Ninety percent of Gunshot wounds to the head are fatal. Most don't even make it to the hospital and those that do have a poor quality of life. I saw blood on President Trump's face, and I was worried about a more severe injury to the brain. I prayed. I was in shock. Trump immediately ducked and then was whisked off stage by the secret service but not before he stood up with blood dripping down his face and shouted, "Fight, Fight, Fight!" with his hands up in the air letting us know he was okay. The country was in shock. President Trump was almost killed.

The bullet's trajectory shifted by the hand of God. What should have been a direct hit became a near miss of death as if a divine hand had intervened, altering the path of the bullet. It was an act that defied all understanding, a testament to the power of God's protection.

In the aftermath, there was a mixture of shock, disbelief, and awe. How could such a precise shot go astray? How could the laws of physics and probability bend in such a manner? The answer, for many, was clear: it was a miracle, a sign of God's protective shield over Donald Trump. I cried. I was at work when I was first notified by Fox. I was up all night reporting on President Trump's injury, his course of medical care and what would unfold in the hospital. It wasn't just a physical injury, but it was also a massive trauma to the soul of our nation. A former President was nearly assassinated but by the grace of God, his life was spared.

Medical professionals, security experts, and bystanders alike were left grappling with the inexplicable nature of what had occurred. The incident became a focal point for discussions on faith, divine intervention, and the miraculous ways in which God works in our lives. This miraculous event serves as a powerful testament to the unwavering faith that many hold. It is a reminder that, even in the face of danger and adversity, God's presence is ever vigilant, watching over us and intervening in ways that transcend human understanding.

In the field of medicine, we often rely on empirical evidence and scientific reasoning to navigate the complexities of life and health. Yet, there are moments when the divine intersects with the mortal, reminding us of the boundless power of faith and the miracles that stem from it. The miracle of God protecting President Donald Trump from being hit by the bullet is a profound illustration of divine intervention in our lives. It reaffirms the belief that, beyond the stethoscope and the realms of human understanding, there exists a higher power guiding and protecting us. As we continue to explore the intersection of faith and medicine, let us remain open to the miracles that unfold around us, recognizing them as manifestations of God's infinite love and protection.

CHAPTER 1

Rage, Fear, Resilience: The City's Unseen War

In the city that never sleeps, where the lights shine brightly, and dreams are as tall as skyscrapers, a different kind of story unfolds—a story that is not often told, not in the glitz and glamour of Broadway or the hustle and bustle of Wall Street. This one happens in the shadows, in the forgotten corners of the city. It's a story of violence, pain, and loss. It's a story about Officer Rivera, Officer Mora, and victims of violence in this city.

Officer Rivera was an honest and hardworking young American. A country boy from Bristol, Tennessee, he went to the police academy to pursue a career he loved and went on to become a respected officer. Life was good. But then, a few months ago, out of nowhere, he was shot several times by an allegedly mentally ill man while responding to a distress call. But before Officer Mora, his partner, could reach his radio and call the incident in, he suffered the same fate as Officer Rivera.

Officers Rivera and Mora were the epitome of courage and dedication. They walked the beat with unwavering resolve, always ready to protect and serve. But their lives were cut tragically short by a mentally ill man who pulled the trigger on that fateful night. Their loss shattered my heart and left me feeling hopeless. Such promising lives were extinguished so needlessly, and it was so preventable.

THE WAVE OF VIOLENCE

This tragedy is not isolated. Violence permeates nearly every corner of the city. One busy evening, the emergency room doors burst open, revealing a distressed man from 42nd Street. His earlobe dangled, almost severed, after an unprovoked attack with a metal bar. I attended to his injuries, meticulously stitching up the wound. As he recovered, he spoke of the random violence that seemed to have gripped the city's soul. My heart sank, but this was just the beginning.

Days later, I treated a senior from East 67th Street. He'd suffered a cracked skull after a brutal mugging. Because of the extent of his injuries, it was a miracle that he survived. His family was grateful for my care, but I wished such atrocities could end.

The trend continued with an Asian gentleman from 69th Street. Tears streamed down his face as he recounted the assault he'd experienced returning from work. The multiple abrasions, bruises, and rib fractures were testaments to the brutality of the attack. As I treated him, I found myself not only healing physical wounds but also offering emotional support.

The scams at 96th Street were perhaps the most sinister. One patient had been deceived into believing he had accidentally injured someone with his vehicle. When he stopped out of concern, he was ambushed and assaulted. Another struck from behind, rendering him unconscious.

HEALING THE DEEP WOUNDS

These stories are a grim testament to the unseen war that rages in our city. They are a call to action, a plea for change. The tragic deaths of Officer Rivera and Officer Mora served as a grim reminder of the consequences of unaddressed mental illness and societal violence. Yet, their legacy can also become an inspiration that can spark a movement that could change the trajectory of a community.

Ezekiel 45:9 urges us to put away violence and destruction. It encourages us to practice justice and righteousness. To have healthy emotional minds, we should expose ourselves to this associated with kindness and goodness. So, we must do better for Officer Rivera, for Officer Mora, and for all the victims who walk through my ER doors every day.

In the city that never sleeps, we cannot afford to turn a blind eye to the war against violence. We must stand up, speak out, and fight for a safer city for all.

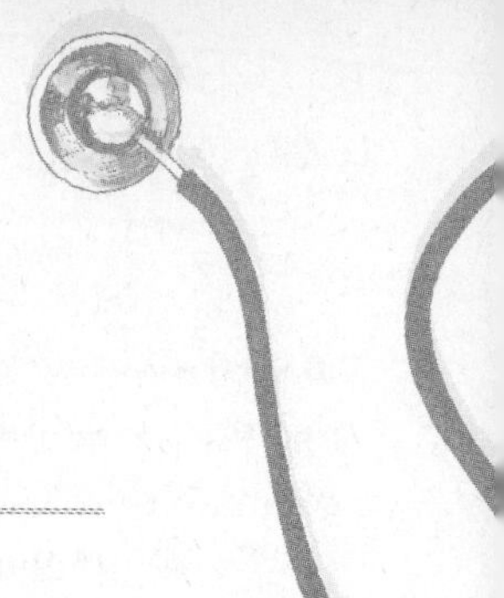

CHAPTER 2

In Between Love and Grief

Art is long, and Time is fleeting,
And our hearts, though stout and brave,
Still, like muffled drums, are beating
Funeral marches to the grave.

—Henry Wadsworth Longfellow (1807–82),
"A Psalm of Life"

America in early 2020 was like someone who was suddenly sucker punched: It was taken by surprise. It had the wind knocked out of it. Anyone who lived in America at the time experienced a palpable sense of confusion as the virus began to spread far and wide within American borders. People toggled between news sources, trying to separate facts from speculation.

The country staggered financially as well; industries ground to a halt due to the devastating economic blow. Businesses shut down, millions lost their jobs, and the stock market plummeted due to the sudden decrease in the value of stocks traded on the stock exchange. This made investors experience substantial financial losses, and in turn, everyone was affected in one way or another. Socially, stay-at-home orders and social distancing measures left streets deserted and cities eerily quiet. The psychological impact these lockdowns had on people was insurmountable—as much as it was for the benefit of everyone, it had very negative effects from person to person based on factors like personality, preexisting mental health conditions, living situation, and available social support.

Hospitals and healthcare facilities found themselves overwhelmed due to the sudden patient surge; hospital resources were strained, from ICU beds to personal protective equipment (PPE), forcing healthcare workers to make difficult choices. I remember overhearing a conversation between a certain woman and her friend in the waiting area of the hospital while filling out some forms at the receptionist's desk. I later treated her and found out her name was Emily. She talked so loudly that even the mask covering her mouth couldn't silence her voice.

"Can you believe all that has been happening lately? Honestly, life has changed so drastically that I am still reeling from the shock of it! I mean, what is all this? We can't even sit within six feet of each other!" Emily exclaimed in exasperation.

"Yeah, it's crazy, isn't it?" the other woman, who I assumed was her friend or maybe someone she knew, responded softly.

"I just can't believe this is happening. I mean, a global pandemic? It sounds like something out of a movie," Emily reiterated.

"I know what you mean. I am not much of a news person. When I started hearing reports of the virus, I thought it would just blow over after a few weeks. It has been months now, and I am unsure about that. It's like we're living in an alternate reality!" she said sadly.

"Exactly! One moment, people are saying it was just a bad flu, and the next minute, the government is talking about lockdowns and quarantines, and we can't leave our houses without wearing masks!" Emily added. Her frustration was evident.

"I understand the frustration, but you know what, God got us. I felt like I would lose my mind, but reading the Bible has been such a great source of solace and strength," the woman said. After a few minutes, her name was called by one of the nurses, and she stood up to leave, but not before leaving her friend with one last word. "I encourage you to read Philippians 4:6–7. It will help with all the anxiety and frustration you are feeling. I wish you the best in your treatment today."

As I stood there, I felt quite hopeful to see that more people were embracing the word of God at these very difficult and confusing times. I had a renewed sense of inspiration from this patient, because if civilians who did not fully understand the depths and impact of this crisis were steadfast in the Lord, what about me as a medical professional and a believer? This was the time to stand strong in my faith and believe all would be fine. When I got to my office, I opened my Bible to read Philippians 4:6–7 KJV. It said:

> Do not be anxious about anything, but
> in every situation, by prayer and petition,
> with thanksgiving, present your requests
> to God. And the peace of God, which
> transcends all understanding, will guard
> your hearts and minds in Christ Jesus.

When I tell you after reading this verse, I felt an unexplainable sense of peace and calmness, I mean it. There was a positive energy about me that flowed to every patient I saw from that point. Apart from trying to treat their various ailments, I encouraged them and reminded them of a power beyond us that was constantly watching over us. When Emily was later called to the room, I gave her hope and encouragement. Everyone needed some hope, understanding, and encouragement during those trying times. We were all struggling in one way or another—some with their health, some with their finances, and others with loneliness and isolation. If you could hold yourself together during this period, it was only prudent to try to comfort and encourage others. For the Bible says in 2 Corinthians 1:3–4 KJV:

> Praise be to the God and Father of our Lord Jesus Christ, the Father of compassion and the God of all comfort, who comforts us in all our troubles so that we can comfort those in any trouble with the comfort we receive from God.

The world is a community of people with lungs and upper respiratory systems that invisible viruses can invade; these viruses can attach themselves to the cells in our lungs and make us very sick. Viruses cannot live independently; they need a host cell to replicate and cause illness. While they are making us sick, they are multiplying in large numbers to infect more people.

There is a process in which viruses multiply and cause illness; it starts with attachment and entry. Viruses often attach themselves to a specific receptor on the surface of a host receptor. Once it does this, it enters the host cell and fuses with the cell membrane. Then, depending on the virus type, it will release its genetic material into the host cell. The genetic material of a virus can either be DNA or RNA. Once the genetic material has been released into the host's body, it will instruct the body's cells to release new viral components that imitate the virus's genetic material, in other words, produce copies of the DNA or RNA of the virus. The latest viral components will then assemble to form complete virus particles called virions. The virus then undergoes structural modification and changes, releasing into the host cells once they mature. Once released, they spread to other cells in the host's body, and the cycle continues.

Some of these viruses are rare or successfully controlled by vaccines developed by science—the polio, smallpox, and measles viruses are three of these. Some of the viruses we have lived with for a very long time, and our bodies have developed defenses that fight off the bad effects fairly well—the coronavirus, for example, is one. The coronavirus causes the common cold, but when it mutates—which it often does when passing through communities of other kinds of mammals—the mutations, also called variants, can invade human respiratory systems in forms our bodies' immune systems do not recognize for the purpose of countering to thwart serious disease. The SARS-CoV-2 virus is one of these mutations, albeit likely engineered in a lab.

When a new variant attacks someone and uses that person for rapid and enormous replication, the infected person can infect another person or many others. Then, the spread grows so quickly and rampantly that vast numbers of people become sickened.

The transmission happened in various ways—infected individuals passed it on to the uninfected mostly through respiratory droplets (like coughing and sneezing). This is why people were advised to avoid face-to-face interactions, wear masks, wash their hands with soap and water, and so forth.

The political divisions quickly started; the response to the virus became a political battleground, with many political leaders addressing the nation and giving their views. Those messages were mostly different because everyone had their own personal opinion on the best ways to combat the virus. The conflicting statements from leaders and deep-seated political divisions hindered a cohesive national strategy, leaving the country unable to respond effectively. Most people aligned themselves with certain political parties and made it into an "us" versus "them" mentality. COVID affected all of us; the divisions only made it harder for people to compromise or find common ground to accommodate everyone's beliefs and solve the problem. Some political leaders' ambition and greed mainly fueled the political divisions. James 3:16 KJV says,

"For where you have envy and selfish ambition, there you find disorder and every evil practice."

But in all, God encourages us to stay united in mind and thought: "I appeal to you, brothers and sisters, in the name of our Lord Jesus Christ, that all of you agree with one another in what you say and that there be no divisions among you, but that you be perfectly united in mind and thought" (1 Corinthians 1:10 NIV).

This is what happened to the world and to the United States in early 2020.

PRAYER

Father Lord, in the midst of all our trials and transgressions, we call upon you to bring peace and understanding in our lives. Lord, without you, we are not worthy of any good thing, but with you, we are worthy of so much more. Give us the heart to always be willing to make compromises to accommodate others and to benefit us all. We come against any power that tries to bring confusion and division among your people, and may we always be led in your faith and honor. Amen.

REFLECTION

Reflecting on how life transformed after the pandemic, we can learn many lessons from this period. How are you practically living out your faith? Is your faith in God beneficial to others? Are you helping people find their strength and renew their hope in Christ? We should apply our faith in day-to-day life. You can be the reason someone feels encouraged and approaches life with a renewed sense of hope. So many people are struggling with battles they may not speak about; spreading love, compassion, and kindness can go a long way in making things better for some people. Speak life into someone today and remind them of the promises and goodness of the Lord. You do not know how many lives a kind word can save.

THE WORLD IN TURMOIL

In the United States, so many people got sick that the economy and societal norms were affected. The damage had two roots. One, sick people could not work and had to isolate themselves from others, including from people who loved them and could care for them. Two, healthy people had to change their behavior—not shopping in stores, not going to restaurants, hair salons, theaters, and the like to avoid becoming sick themselves and becoming agents of virus transmission. These two community shocks rocked our economy and society emotionally, spiritually, and socially.

I had a patient who took to shopping as a form of therapy, so you can imagine how hard it was to be in a stressful environment and not be able to do the thing that affords you some release or happiness. One might think she was just vain, and she used shopping as an excuse to hoard and buy more things. As a medical professional, I have come to understand the psychology behind shopping or gambling not only as a form of stress relief but also as an addiction. Shopping temporarily shifts focus away from stressors, and the excitement of new purchases can trigger feelings of happiness and pleasure. Additionally, choosing items and making decisions provides a sense of control—a control nobody had during the time of COVID. Quarantine and lockdown were very hard on her, so she kept herself sedated and intoxicated most of the time because she had no outlet to deal with the realities of life. I am only glad family surrounded her at the time, as her mental health was still greatly affected and deteriorated. I know of people who are not so lucky to have that kind of support from their families. Most were neglected during their times of need and could not get the help they needed. God encourages families to always stand by and support each other whenever someone needs it. Those who do not support their families are admonished even in the Bible: "Anyone who does not provide for their relatives, and especially for their own household, has denied the faith and is worse than an unbeliever" (1 Timothy 5:8 NIV).

Not being able to go to work was a huge problem. Fortunately for our economy, current technology allowed millions of workers to do their jobs online from home. Because so many people have jobs that are done through the internet anyway, all one needed was a good connection and good Wi-Fi, and they could work from bedrooms, kitchens, and dining rooms as well as they could at an office. But for many people, the workplace or office was where they spent most of their day and interacted most with people, including friends, mentors, and people they admired. Suddenly, those people and social interactions disappeared and reappeared via computer screens. Gone was the irritating commute, but also gone was wholesome human contact. Humans thrive on social engagement. Loneliness is a medical hazard.

At first, working remotely felt like an answered prayer for many because then they could stay home and not worry about the hustle and bustle of getting to work and the long hours usually spent in traffic. But soon, the isolation and loneliness started to creep in, especially for people living alone or those who valued in-person interactions with their colleagues. Those families found it hard to have a work-life balance, because if you're doing all your work at home, at what point do you disconnect and become a present parent? The boundaries between life and work became a blur. Some people spent too much time on work, or they spent too little—these extreme variables brought issues either with the family or with their jobs. There were also many distractions at home for obvious reasons; most homes don't have a conducive environment for work. Between household chores and personal and parental responsibilities, there was just too much going on to focus solely on work. Many fell behind on their deadlines and ended up getting retrenched.

Statistics also show that staying at home compounded marital problems, and divorce cases were at an all-time high. Imagine having husbands and wives who did not generally spend twenty-four hours a day together. All of a sudden, these people were confined to their houses or apartments with the same person day after day, month after month. The proximity and constant interaction led to disagreements and conflicts over minor issues compounded by the heightened stress and frustration of everything happening in the world. With both partners at home, most families experienced the pressure of equal domestic responsibilities. An imbalance in household chores and childcare responsibilities led to resentment. The absence of personal space and alone time also made it challenging to recharge and maintain individual identities separate from their roles as husband and wife. People lost themselves, and miscommunications or assumptions about each other's needs and expectations arose, causing misunderstandings. The increased conflict caused friction, conflict, trouble, and, in worst-case scenarios, led to murder.

This was a miserable period for some families; that is why the Bible constantly teaches love among families so that in times of difficulties, their love for each other can help them weather the storms. Without the love of God in our families, many homes will not stand.

"Love is patient, love is kind. It does not envy, it does not boast, it is not proud. It does not dishonor others, it is not self-seeking, it is not easily angered, and it keeps no record of wrongs. Love does not delight in evil but rejoices with the truth. It always protects, always trusts, always hopes, and always perseveres" (1 Corinthians 13:4–7 NIV).

Ephesians 4:2–3 NIV further underscores this message by telling us, "Be completely humble and gentle; be patient, bearing with one another in love. Make every effort to keep the unity of the Spirit through the bond of peace."

Children, too, were suddenly at home twenty-four hours a day. They felt just as cooped up and anxious because they could not be in school or play with other children. Adding more to the stress of kids staying home and not going to school meant parents were now responsible for their children's education, getting them in front of computer screens at the proper time, and making sure they stayed focused on lessons. Zoom became a new household word.

These 24/7 responsibilities became challenging situations for many people. Everyone needs a break sometime; everyone needs some private time. But the new normal of staying at home brought a lot of socioeconomic problems and real stress into people's lives. There developed a high incidence of domestic violence, suicide, homicide, child neglect, and abuse.

The cases of child neglect and abuse are probably the ones that tore my heart the most. I want to say that some parents were going through a lot and could not be there entirely for their children, but still, there is no excuse for abuse and neglect. I heard of a case where a child was only given water and two slices of bread daily while the pantry was stocked up with food just because the mother was extremely paranoid about food and ending up being unable to get some. This child was literally starving and getting malnourished by the day. Thankfully, a good and kind neighbor came to the rescue and even got the child treated at our hospital.

Children born into violent families also suffered the most because now all the frustrations about what was going on in the world were being taken out on them. Those who would be physically abused maybe once every week were now at the hands of their oppressors each day and every hour. I do not even want to talk about the kids being sexually abused at home by people they trusted; COVID-19 only compounded their woes. It broke my heart how much suffering befell most children, because children are one of the most valued people in the kingdom of God. They should be treated with kindness, protected, loved, and cared for, yet they suffered the most. They were the lowest risk population when it came to COVID complications but were hurt the most with school closures, lockdowns, and being forced to wear masks. And as a result, we now see children behind in education, speech, growth, and developmental milestones with an increase of ER visits for mental health ailments among children who presented with anxiety and suicidal ideation.

The Bible says in Mark 10:13–16 NIV, "People were bringing little children to Jesus for him to place his hands on them, but the disciples rebuked them. When Jesus saw this, he was indignant. He said to them, 'Let the little children come to me, and do not hinder them, for the kingdom of God belongs to such as these.'"

In my practice as a doctor, I could see the troubles this new normal was causing. And it was not only the stress of dealing with partners and children at home. There were serious health issues as people became less active. They sat in their rooms and hardly moved around. People became depressed, overweight, and even obese. I could see this from those who came into our healthcare facility complaining of medical troubles such as diabetes, heart disease, and depression. Cancer screenings were missed. Dentist visits and basic childhood immunizations fell behind. Oral health is linked to heart health, and heart disease is still the number one killer in this country for both men and women.

COVID brought with it a lot of respiratory complications such as pneumonia and acute respiratory distress syndrome (ARDS), especially to people who were immunocompromised. The cardiovascular complications included myocarditis, pericarditis, and blood clots. It was a difficult period for people who suffered from heart disease and ran the risk of blood clots for various reasons. One of the earliest symptoms of COVID included loss of taste and smell. Many people joked around about this symptom, but it was only funny when you were not experiencing it. Some individuals experienced brain fog, memory problems, and, in worst-case scenarios, strokes or pulmonary embolisms resulting in sudden death.

Overall, COVID-19 greatly impacted people's health and well-being; this is when people realized that the accurate measure of wealth is health. Many people with money could afford the best medicine and medical doctors that money could provide, yet they still perished at the hands of COVID. Money could not provide relief; only God can help us: "He said, 'If you listen carefully to the LORD your God and do what is right in his eyes, if you pay attention to his commands and keep all his decrees, I will not bring on you any of the diseases I brought on the Egyptians, for I am the LORD, who heals you'" (Exodus 15:26 NIV).

Even when people did get out of their homes and apartments for errands, or whatever they needed to do, the human interactions they were once used to and that could boost their spirits were far from rewarding. COVID dictated that hugging and touching were forbidden. Grandparents died alone because of social isolation restrictions. Because of masks, we could not see smiles or expressions of any sort. All we could see were eyes. It was as if we were dealing with bandits trying to hide their identities. This was detrimental to good mental health, an important ingredient in good physical health.

Physically, life did not change much for me. Like healthcare professionals around the country, I had to keep going to work no matter what to treat others and counter this disease. I often thought of my family, especially my mom, as I walked home from work through Times Square and saw it empty, so quiet, with no human sounds. It was like out of a science fiction movie. Times Square was deserted! It was unreal.

But then, of course, the economy had to go on, people had to do their jobs, or food would not be on grocery store shelves, electricity and fuel for heat would not be delivered, and trash could not be collected. So, people in their apartments and houses sporadically appeared on the streets again. Since we all had to learn how to live with this disease, it amazed me the creativity of humans in the face of problems. Suddenly, masks of all sorts cropped up: designer masks, rhinestone masks, superhero masks, funny and cultural masks. It was good to see people pushing back in the face of adversity.

Things also changed at my workplace. How healthcare providers interacted with patients changed and not for the better. We looked strange as we wore PPE, and it was a bit awkward for us to even move about, which must have been off-putting for patients. We were surrounded by disease all day long; we had to be careful around patients. This was not our normal way of working with people. A lot of doctor-patient interaction depends on trust. We doctors have to trust that our patients are telling us the complete truth about their symptoms and behaviors, or we are liable to make a misdiagnosis or get sick.

Conversely, we doctors must demonstrate that we are trustworthy, that we will not divulge our patients' medical conditions to anyone without their permission, and that we are super careful with their most intimate communications. We take an oath to be so. Accordingly, we must show empathy and work to create a relationship of confidence. Wearing weird astronaut PPE and standing back do not lend themselves to creating such a relationship. We created barriers between doctor and patient that nobody in my profession liked.

All this new normal made life uncertain because there was not much we could do about being forced to apply the protection guidelines or the precaution procedures on how we must be guarded against people. A virus and not a bacterium caused this pandemic. Antibiotics can work on bacteria but not on viruses. We could prescribe painkillers and cough medicine, and we could give inhalers to people who were short of breath. But that was about it. And in the beginning, people were fearful. They knew about COVID-19 and what it could do. Especially in New York City, where I worked, a horrific number of people in the spring of 2020 were dying; the morgues were full, and patients wondered, "Am I going to die?" It was all very distressing for both people who were sick and for us in the healthcare field.

The old normal was definitely broken. The new normal was bad, and it continued to be bad. Our federal government had a chance to make things better but failed. The government had the opportunity to plan for new variants but did not use the Defense Production Act when omicron hit to ramp up manufacturing for new tests and medications. The nation's citizens were told the administration would be ready, but this turned out to be just words. They failed.

The administration should have had billions of COVID tests ready to go. They should have had stockpiles of medications and antivirals ready to go. They should have allowed the use of off label medications that could have saved lives. But doctors were threatened with losing their license and were censured if we did so. We had medications like Paxlovid available in high quantities. Paxlovid is not a substitute for the vaccines, but it does help to slow down SARS-CoV-2 in the body. The same goes for monoclonal antibody treatments. Again, these are not substitutes for vaccines, but they helped in healing. Medicine became political. We should not have been fighting over what drugs to use when we were fighting to save lives. The federal government learned about the effectiveness of these treatments but waited too long to ramp them up.

The failure of our federal, state, and local governments to be ready with tests and medicines was dire. When the wave of the delta variant hit in the summer of 2021, people lined up for miles and had to wait three and four hours to be tested. It was utterly unacceptable.

The government was unprepared for delta. Officials should have seen it coming. In the spring of 2021, four thousand people a day were dying from delta in India, where this variant developed. As soon as it was carried to the United States, officials should have known it was going to mushroom and it did. Lots of people were caught unaware.

Good news came in the early summer of 2021 when the vaccines became widespread because of the success of Operation Warp Speed. COVID cases were declining, but then, boom—the delta virus surfaced and was so lethal that even people who had been vaccinated and boosted were getting breakthrough cases of COVID.

The administration should have learned lessons from the time of the delta variant to be ready for other variants. But then the omicron variant hit hard late in 2021, and the same troubles cropped up. Did we not learn our lesson? There were not enough tests; there were long lines and long waiting times for being tested; there were not enough medicines that could relieve symptoms; and there were confusing policies about wearing masks, social distancing, gathering in groups, and allowing children to go to school. All of this was bad for adults and children mentally, emotionally, and nutritionally.

Even funerals, with all their attendant grief, were adversely affected by this pandemic. At the cemetery, people were not allowed to get out of their cars, and only the immediate family could get out of their cars when the casket was lowered into the ground. Some bereaved could only mourn via live streams. But when the streaming was over, everything disappeared as if everyone and everything weren't there anymore. Because of COVID, people couldn't touch, feel, or hug. They couldn't give condolences. They were cut off from people. Humanity and dignity were also dead.

As if grief was not the only painful emotion, the restrictions on funeral processions added more to the grief and sadness, making it even harder on families. But as believers, people still had so much hope and faith in the wonders that God can do even in death: "Brothers and sisters, we do not want you to be uninformed about those who sleep in death so that you do not grieve like the rest of mankind, who have no hope. For we believe that Jesus died and rose again, and so we believe that God will bring with Jesus those who have fallen asleep in him" (1 Thessalonians 4:13–14 NIV).

Jesus further tells us that those who died in Christ will be resurrected with him: "Jesus said to her, 'I am the resurrection and the life. The one who believes in me will live, even though they die, and whoever lives by believing in me will never die. Do you believe this?'" (John 11:25–26 NIV).

And if you do not believe this, believe that there is a better place waiting for us on the other side, a life free from the troubles and sorrows of the world. Jesus promised us that he has gone ahead to prepare a better place for all who believe in him and his father: "Do not let your hearts be troubled. You believe in God; believe also in me. My Father's house has many rooms; if that were not so, would I have told you that I am going there to prepare a place for you? And if I go and prepare a place for you, I will come back and take you to be with me that you also may be where I am." (John 14:1–3 NIV).

PRAYER

Lord, now more than ever, the family unit needs you. We seek your guidance and protection over our families. May you be the head and help keep the love among your children. Protect all the children in the world from abuse and neglect, and may you direct their destiny helpers to them. Receive the souls of our departed loved ones who died in your mercy and give them rest. Amen.

REFLECTION

In this reflection, we focus on the family unit; marriage and family are no longer what they used to be. So many marriages are breaking apart because people do not take their vows seriously and are unwilling to work to make their marriages a success. There is a great need for compassion and tolerance in marriages, and people must make compromises because nobody is 100 percent perfect. Focus on the good in each other instead of dwelling on the negative. Parents, it is your duty to love and protect children; children, it is your duty to obey and respect your parents.

GRAPPLING WITH THE AFTEREFFECTS OF COVID-19

So much of what we knew of life before COVID has gone away and horrendously changed. I was living with my sister in New York

City but was worried; I didn't want to get her sick. She moved to Nashville as I was mingling with the virus my whole long working day, and I wouldn't have been able to bear it if I had brought it home and seen her catch it. I also decided I wouldn't visit my mother in Tennessee until things calmed down. I stayed away from her for a few months, and when I finally got to see her, I wore a mask, fearing I would contaminate her since I was around COVID all day long treating sick patients.

One of my colleagues got COVID and suffered neurological and kidney damage. When I called him one day, he started crying. He was so grateful to hear from me. So many of these patients were pushed to their limits of mental and emotional stamina. Even the young ones, people in the prime of their lives, non-smokers, were having huge problems like chest pain and difficulty breathing.

Some medical facilities had to shut down because many medical staff were sick. And, of course, this is exactly what you don't want: fewer medical facilities when a pandemic is going on. The result is sick people being unable to get a diagnosis, counseling, and treatment they need.

The whole healthcare system was destroyed, if not forced to a standstill. Naturally, we who worked in locations to which all these COVID-sick people came were very vulnerable to becoming infected ourselves. We were on the front lines in the trenches with so much high risk. Most of the time—at least at the facility where I work the most—we were very lucky to have had all the PPE we required. At the time, President Trump sent us the USNS *Comfort* for added support. Watching it dock here in the city was symbolic of the immense support we needed and received. Still, vast numbers of healthcare workers became sick despite being fully aware of how the disease spreads and what it can do to the body, and, of course, some of them died. It has been tragic, and these frontline people have been heroes. They know the risks and expose themselves to the virus daily, day after day after day. It wears you down mentally, and because of the mental wear, you suffer physical wear. And when you have both mental and physical wear, you are more likely to contract the virus and more likely to suffer harshly from it.

The healthcare facility staffing shortage became very real and very burdensome. It still is. One result is that patients wait longer to see a doctor or nurse. They are sick, in bad moods, and ache with pain. It's no wonder some of them are impatient and rude. At our healthcare facility, a patient's most common complaint is: "I had to wait too long." Of course, they think it's okay because their bodies ache so badly, but many act poorly, complain too much, or don't use proper judgment. Some should go to a hospital emergency room rather than an urgent care center, and some should go to the doctors they already have. But they don't; they come to our facility. Some are extremely kind and understanding, some inconsiderate. We do the best we can. We're polite. We're sympathetic. But we are also human. Sometimes, we put in fourteen- to fifteen-hour days. We are exhausted at the end of each shift. I would go home with throbbing aching feet from standing all day and on top of that always wondered if that was the day I would catch COVID myself.

Sometimes, one thoughtful remark can make up for thirty unkind ones, especially when some of our patients are sincerely concerned for us. They ask how we are holding up and if we are well. They thank us for what we do and tell us they know how hard we work. I would receive supportive emails and messages from viewers, patients, and colleagues, which was so inspiring and motivating. That really helps. It's such a small thing to show they care, and it really helped our morale. Proverbs 16:24 KJV says, "Gracious words are like a honeycomb, sweetness to the soul and health to the body."

Children, especially, have been badly affected and deprived. I believe the schools could have operated safely. They should not have been shut down. Keeping kids at home with remote learning is a far cry from in-class interaction and learning. These are precious learning years that impact children for life. Evidently, staying at home was also bad on another important level. Reports have shown that staying at home from school and the absent interactions and canceled school activities added to the anxiety, stress, and depression in children that often resulted in many cases of attempted and actual suicide.

PRAYER

Dear Lord, grant us the wisdom to see beyond differences and to treat every person we encounter with respect and compassion. Fill our hearts with empathy so we may understand their struggles and offer a listening ear and a helping hand. May my words always be kind, and may you help us overcome our selfishness.

REFLECTION

Kindness is one of the best Christian virtues anyone can have. You will come across many opportunities to show somebody kindness; it can be as simple as a call to check up on how they're doing, buying someone food, reading the word of God to them, or being kind in your speech. It is always important to appreciate the people who offer us a service, regardless of whether it is their job. A simple thank you goes a long way.

SYSTEMIC STRUGGLES INTENSIFIED: COVID-19'S UNEQUAL TOLL ON MARGINALIZED COMMUNITIES

We cannot fail to shed light on the devastating impact of COVID on marginalized communities. It hurt minority and marginalized communities harder than the better-off ones because we found that COVID kills more in minority and marginalized communities. COVID puts more people in those communities out of work. Depriving them of income that was the lowest in the country to begin with didn't help.

A Brookings Institution study early in the pandemic showed that Black and Hispanic/Latino death rates were six times higher than for whites and that Blacks were shown to be dying at a rate higher than whites ten years older. These trends have persisted ever since.

Detailed investigations of why this is so are yet to be completed. Still, the reasons are very likely ones already surmised:. Blacks and Hispanics/Latinos have a higher rate of health problems to begin with—diabetes, hypertension, obesity, and lung disease—and thus have more serious outcomes when they contract COVID; they have less access to health care on account of having lower rates of health insurance than whites; many live in communities where people are more densely compact. Many work jobs that require their presence, and many work in areas that are more likely to harbor the SARS-CoV-2 virus, namely hospitals and nursing homes. The death rates are mirrored in the rates of people sickened but surviving.

In addition, Blacks and Hispanics/Latinos have lower vaccination rates than whites (see reports by the Kaiser Family Foundation, among others), though Hispanics/Latinos are catching up to whites. Since the appearance of vaccines in 2021, it has been shown that vaccinated people are far less likely to become seriously ill from COVID and even much less likely to die from the disease.

This is good. And it also bears repeating that with respect to the egregious Tuskegee syphilis scandal of the 1930s and 1940s, Black men were not injected with the syphilis bacterium. Rather, in order to study the progression of the disease for which there was no known cure at the time, some Blacks who already had syphilis were *not* given penicillin when it became available in 1947. This shameful episode certainly casts shame on the government, but it in no way demonstrates that the privately developed (by Pfizer, Moderna, and Johnson & Johnson) vaccines are not the effective virus-fighting medicines they are or that the government is in some way deliberately trying to sicken large portions of the nation's population.

PRAYER

Almighty God, we pray for marginalized communities worldwide. In these challenging times, they bear the brunt of numerous burdens, and I ask for your compassion and healing touch to be upon them. Please give them the strength and resilience to fight against systemic injustices. And above all, shower your blessings upon them and eliminate all health disparities. Amen.

REFLECTIONS

How often do you watch an injustice to a minority and keep quiet? Have you been your brother's or sister's advocate? As a believer in the almighty, we are called to be advocates of the Lord to our brothers and sisters. When you keep quiet about an injustice being done to a minority, you become part of the problem. Stand up not only for yourself but for those who do not have the strength to do that for themselves. If you are in a position of power or advantage, use it to help others. Stand up for everyone irrespective of their race, gender, religion, or ethnic group, just like God is for all of us.

RISING TO THE CHALLENGE: OVERCOMING PERSONAL OBSTACLES DURING THE COVID-19 PANDEMIC

I am a survivor, and after conquering the pandemic, I have not been a stranger to hardship or circumstances that forced me to adapt, fight off demons, and push forward for a better world for myself, my family, and others. I had to leave a good normal for a bad new normal, and I made the new normal work for me.

Personally, the hardest time for me and my family was the passing of my father when I was thirteen years old. We lived in a small community in central Florida where my father worked as a chemist with the Lake County Pollution Control Department, while my mom was a nurse at Harry-Anna Children's Hospital (also known as the Florida Elks Children's Hospital). My parents were immigrants who came to this country from the war-torn Middle East to find the American dream. We all loved living in a state where it was summer all year, on an orange grove where it was fun and safe to run around. My mother would do the dishes at the kitchen sink and look out the window to see us playing in the field. She didn't have to worry about us being kidnapped or run down by a car.

My widowed mom took care of us, four girls and one boy, and sacrificed to provide for our needs, especially to ensure we completed our education. I will also be forever grateful to my mom for bringing us up in faith; she laid a moral and ethical foundation that has forever shaped my values in life. I better understood right from wrong from when I was still a child. Knowing God helped me to find a sense of purpose and belonging even when nothing seemed to make sense in my life after my father died. Being part of the church gave me a sense of community and belonging, which, as the daughter of immigrant parents, I highly needed. I have been guided by the wisdom and teachings of God my whole life; every time I felt like I was losing a sense of direction, I turned back to the Bible. And not once has it ever failed me. I have recognized the blessings in my life and express gratitude and contentment for them. Faith helps people to focus and appreciate what they have rather than always striving for more without appreciation. It has also broadened my perspective; I do not dwell on the troubles of now but on the goodness of the Lord that is to come. More families should strive to raise their children in faith and with the knowledge of the word of God. "These commandments that I give you today are to be on your hearts. Impress them on your children. Talk about them when you sit at home, walk along the road, lie down, and get up" (Deuteronomy 6:6–7 KJV).

This Bible verse is further reiterated in Psalm 78:4–6 KJV: "We will not hide them from their descendants; we will tell the next generation the praiseworthy deeds of the Lord, his power, and the wonders he has done. He decreed statutes for Jacob and established the law in Israel, which he commanded our ancestors to teach their children so that the next generation would know them, even the children yet to be born, and they, in turn, would tell their children."

Mom also became a nurse for our parish (school nurse, more so). She did blood pressure screenings in the church. She often drove us children to community service events. That's where we learned about community service, about giving back. I think that's when I began to look around and really look closely at other people to see if they needed help. I felt like I wanted them to be all right, to be content.

Looking back on it, I think we as a family—my mother in the lead—worked to make the calamity of my father's death a tragic lesson by which to learn and grow, to turn a negative into a positive. As a family, we set our minds to that and it worked. We became strong.

My mother inspired me to be a doctor, and eventually, I entered medical school. It was tough. Medical school is difficult for everyone. There's a tremendous amount of material to absorb and memorize. You're studying all the time. It's almost crushing in a way. I can remember crying sometimes, worrying about how hard it was and wanting to do well. I prayed a lot, prayed to stay focused, and to keep working hard. There was only one way to deal with medical school: perseverance and hard work. I knew those two things, did them, and got through. I got my medical degree.

Then came residency, and that was hard in a different way. The hours are very long, and you work very hard and are still learning on the job. You are also called on to make medical choices for patients. And that can be daunting as a beginner. I wanted to do well and do my best, especially when performing procedures such as intubation, or a lumbar puncture, or delivering a baby, or facing a circumstance when a patient stopped breathing, but my mother reminded me that in the first year of residency, I would usually have an experienced doctor with me and God by my side to provide the best care possible for my patients. She was right.

In my second year of residency, I remember delivering a baby. The baby's head was stuck. Well, this was not good. I could see the baby's face beginning to turn blue, which meant not enough oxygen was getting to her, and her heart rate was dropping. In other words, it was life-threatening. The doctor who was meant to be with me had left the room, and though I thought he would be back soon, he was searching for the attending obstetrician.

There was nothing for me to do except improvise. I wiggled my hand around the baby to the position where her shoulder was stuck. I got her out with no harm to the baby or the mother, but it was a terrifying situation. My heart was pounding inside, yet I stayed calm on the exterior. Every minute mattered. At a time like that, you must remain calm and stay focused, think of your training, use common sense, and do your best.

I've tried to do that ever since.

PRAYER

Almighty ever-loving Father, we humbly pray for this strength and the resilience to rise above our challenges in life. Give us an unyielding spirit, unwavering determination, and unending courage as we navigate the troubles of life. Help us to learn, grow, and transform in the face of adversity and come out the other end victorious. Amen.

REFLECTION

Reflecting on my life challenges, I have realized that sometimes obstacles are a part of God's plan to shape and strengthen our faith. Look at them as an opportunity for growth, to draw closer to God, and to discover yourself. Always trust in God's plan. Proverbs 3:5–6 teaches us to trust in the Lord with all our heart and lean not on our own understanding. You may not see what the Lord is doing now, but His goodness will surely be revealed in time.

My mother would sometimes teach the gospel of forgiveness to me and my siblings when we struggled. Luke 6:37 NIV says, "Do not judge and you will not be judged. Do not condemn, and you will not be condemned. Forgive, and you will be forgiven." She would have us read from the scripture at bedtime to help us not harden our hearts. Colossians 3:13 NIV was also a great help during this period to "bear with each other and forgive one another if any of you has a grievance against someone. Forgive as the Lord forgave you."

PRAYER

Dear Lord, we pray that you may give us the strength to overcome the pain, trauma, and tragedies that lay heavy in our hearts and minds. Help us to heal from the things that deeply wound us. Above all, give us the fortitude to forgive those who have inflicted the wounds and pains on us. Help us let go of any grudge that prevents us from experiencing your love fully.

REFLECTION

Sorrow, anguish, and pain can throw you into a deep, dark place. Life is full of many mysteries, and sometimes certain events come along and shatter your world completely. Yet in the depths of this anguish, in the midst of your pain, the Lord is promising you that if you walk the journey of faith and forgiveness, He will transform your life completely. I realized holding on to pain, fear, or sadness was only harmful. I needed to release the pain, but I didn't know how. Turning to the word of God was the turning point of my life; the powerful message of love radiated through the teachings of Jesus Christ. I realized that faith was not a sign of weakness but an act of spiritual strength and resilience. It helped me to overcome chains of sadness or bitterness that threatened to consume me. Trusting in the Lord and His divine plan has helped me understand the true essence of Christ's love and has helped me and transformed my life.

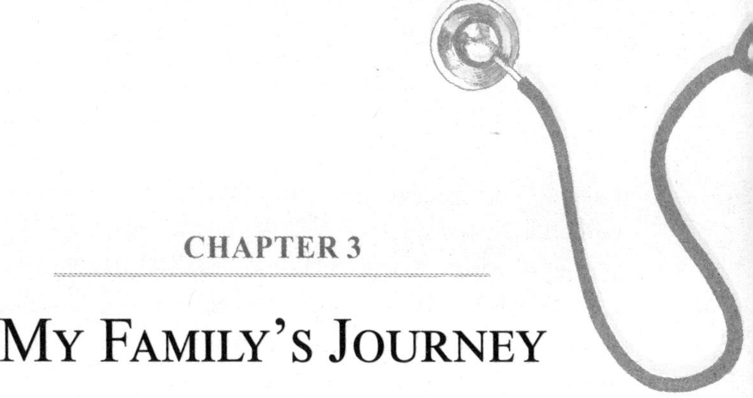

CHAPTER 3

MY FAMILY'S JOURNEY

My story is nothing without family; the essence of my being has been rooted in the family that made me. The journey to becoming who I am could never have been possible without my lovely and supportive family. I am the daughter of immigrant parents who came here searching for the American dream. I am also a first-generation Jordanian American, a fact I am quite proud of. The country of Jordan is home to some of the oldest Christian communities in the world, not to mention biblical sites. A few honorable mentions include Bethany—believed to be the site of Jesus's baptism; there is also the Madaba Mosaic Map, Mount Nebo, and the place is also a beloved pilgrimage destination. I am proud to have my roots in a country with historical Christian communities and diverse denominations. Unfortunately, civil wars erupted in the 1950s, forcing my mother, Hayat, and father, Ben Ziad, to leave Jordan as children with their families. My mother told me how the power struggles and regional conflicts brought about political instability. I remember being very curious about the civil wars that made my parents leave their home country.

"So, what brought the war, Momma?" I asked my mother one afternoon while we sat on our porch.

"Well, we had a king who ruled Jordan. His name was King Abdullah I. Sadly, there were people within his government and different political factions that wanted to curtail his authority," my mother explained.

"Then what happened? Did they succeed?" I asked.

"When the king found out, he dissolved his government and declared martial law. This meant that power was controlled by the military government. This did not please most of the political factions that wanted to gain more influence. So as retaliation, they assassinated the king who started a big crisis in the country," mother explained.

"Is that why you had to leave immediately?" I inquired further.

"Well, not immediately. The crisis led to further political, religious, and economic challenges, which made it harder to live in Jordan. My grandfather was a grocer by trade, and as work became scarce and tensions rose, the family saw that fresh opportunity could be found in America."

"Will we ever go back to Jordan? I would love to see the country where you were born," I said.

"Maybe one day we can visit when you are much older, but not to live. Everything we have is here in America," mother answered with a smile.

That day I couldn't help thinking how hard it must have been for them to find their place in a new country. I came to learn that my mother's father had come to New York ahead of the family, sending for her, her mother, and her two brothers and three sisters once he was established. They arrived in New York aboard the Italian steamer, the SS *Conte Biancamano*.

They had spent twenty-one days below decks.

"To my four-year-old eyes, the Biancamano was the Titanic," my mother said. "I recall scents of vanilla hand soap and eating hard-boiled eggs—smells that I forever associate now with that trip. But we weren't housed above deck, and the journey made many people sick. I couldn't wait to get to New York."

THE NESHEIWATS' TALE OF SURVIVAL AND REDEMPTION

But when they arrived in America, a new set of obstacles awaited. "It was chaotic," my mother often recalled. "People in strange clothes and speaking a foreign language."

The language barrier was perhaps one of the biggest obstacles my mother encountered; she only knew how to communicate in the official language of Jordan, which was Arabic. They only met a few people in New York who understood Arabic, so communication was such a challenge, and they often had to communicate through signs. This was why she desperately wanted to attend kindergarten with her older siblings, so she could learn how to speak English well, but the school sent her home because she was much younger and never understood anything the teacher said.

My mother informed me that this was the first time she experienced rejection, and the whole experience made her feel dejected. Her parents made her understand that schools were much stricter in America, and if she wanted a spot in the school, she would have to prove herself. She was determined to learn as much English as she could in the period she was home such that by the time she went back to school, they wouldn't send her away. Her favorite way to learn English was through television. All she did was repeat everything she heard on the TV, and this helped her improve her pronunciation. She did not know half of what those words meant but was just contented to know how to say them. She would also press her older siblings after school to tell her everything they learned that day. Her aggressiveness towards learning English was one of the reasons she was able to gain basic proficiency quickly.

When she did make it to school a year later, it was heaven: books, a sympathetic teacher, friends, snack time—it was everything she had hoped school would be and more. My mother told me she faced her own fair share of bullying in school. It was horrible being a young, quirky girl from Jordan in New York—the few English words she knew, she spoke with an Arabic accent. The kids would mimic how she said the words and laugh in her face. Sometimes, they would make fun of her cultural clothing. It also didn't help that she had a warm, olive-toned complexion; most of the kids in her class were white except for two other students. She, however, was not going to let anyone kill her buzz. She took all the mean comments in stride and pushed through the negativity. Her mother had instilled in her the virtue of loving your enemies, even those who hurt you. She would always read to her Luke 6:27–29 NIV whenever she came home crying.

> But to you who are listening I say: Love your enemies, do good to those who hate you, bless those who curse you, pray for those who mistreat you. If someone slaps you on one cheek, turn to them the other also. If someone takes your coat, do not withhold your shirt from them.

When the kids realized she was indifferent to all the hateful things they did to her, they ultimately eased up on the bullying. Thankfully, she had a wonderful teacher who tried her best to reprimand the bullies and help her with her studies.

Faith kept the family grounded and involved in Yonkers' vibrant Jordanian community, where my mother and her family worshipped at a church that welcomed all faithful. Community leader (and Human Rights Watch commissioner) George Nassar picked up kids each week for Bible study; the preaching and sermons were a great source of comfort and strength. Times were pretty hard back then; my grandfather was working low income jobs, which sometimes made it difficult to cover most expenses. He had to work three jobs just to sustain the family, not to mention that New York is known for its high cost of living. It was difficult to afford decent housing. They had to live in small, crowded spaces. My mother told me they never felt disillusioned because of their state; they knew things would get better with time. The Lord they served would not let them suffer in abject poverty. Jeremiah 29:11 NIV says, "For I know the plans I have for you, declares the Lord, plans to prosper you and not to harm you, plans to give you hope and a future."

Faith remains a major part of our lives, and I believe that more people should embrace religion to be healthier and feel more stable when the going gets tough.

My mother worked hard in school and really enjoyed studying. She made good friends in school and excelled academically and socially. She was motivated by the desire to live a better life than her parents and provide her children with a better life than she had. She knew that education was going to make all that possible, so she wasn't going to waste the opportunity she had. This was her motto throughout elementary school, junior high school, high school, and college.

My mom became a nurse, my dad a chemist. When their families met and introduced the young Hayat and Ben to each other, my mom and dad quickly fell in love, married, and started their family. In the middle of a hot New York summer, I was born, the second of five children, but we grew up in a small town one hour north of Orlando. My parents moved our large family to Florida where they loved agriculture, and the weather was summer all year round. The Nesheiwat household hummed with activity. Taekwondo, cheerleading, sports, beauty pageants—each child had a distinct interest, traits that would follow us through adulthood. From vacations to the Florida beaches, dinners at Red Lobster, and Sundays at church, I recall my memories of family and faith growing up in Umatilla, Florida, and how those formative years led me to pursue a career healing others.

From the time I was young, I knew I had to work twice as hard as the other students if I wanted to be taken seriously. Sometimes, I was profiled in school because of my appearance, my cultural background, and economic status. I came from a family with very humble beginnings, and this motivated me to double my efforts to exceed expectations and prove people wrong. I was lucky to have the backing of wonderful teachers who, upon noticing my zeal for studies, had taken it upon themselves to ensure I always had the materials I needed to succeed and took me under their wings, especially Mr. Trosper, who taught me how to dissect frogs, and Mrs. Fisher, who taught me how to write. I will never forget them. Because my teachers believed in me, I worked exceptionally hard and was always the top student in my class. I bagged many different awards throughout the course of my studies.

I was not the only one who faced adversities when we made the move to Florida; working as a nurse with a foreign name was at times difficult for my mom. She sometimes experienced unpleasantries from her colleagues being a foreigner and having five kids.

This was all hurtful to my mother, but one thing about her was she would never respond to evil with evil. She knew that the Lord would fight battles for her, for He says in Psalm 12:5 NIV,

"Because the poor are plundered and the needy groan, I will now arise. I will protect them from those who malign them."

She treated even those who maligned her name with kindness. She was polite and respectful, and her patients adored her. She killed everyone with kindness and worked twice as hard at her job because she believed all these challenges could be overcome through kindness. Her good deeds made a difference. The book of 1 Peter 2:9–23 NIV says, "For it is commendable if someone bears up under the pain of unjust suffering because they are conscious of God. But how is it to your credit if you receive a beating for doing wrong and endure it? But if you suffer for doing good and you endure it, this is commendable before God. To this you were called, because Christ suffered for you, leaving you an example, that you should follow in his steps. 'He committed no sin, and no deceit was found in his mouth.' When they hurled their insults at him, he did not retaliate; when he suffered, he made no threats. Instead, he entrusted himself to him who judges justly."

Mom's hard work and resilience and heart full of the love of Christ made our family happy.

PRAYER

Father Lord, we thank you for the gift of family; we thank you for the gift of friendship and all the people we love. Thank you, God, for the way you manifest yourself in our families, for our daily provisions, and also for always making a way, even where there seems to be no way. Jesus Christ, you suffered so that I can be saved; may this salvation always walk with us, and may everyone who encounters us experience your goodness through us. Amen.

REFLECTION

Family is a foundational unit of the church; it is where forgiveness, redemption, and love can flourish. God has given to us the gift of family so that we can experience love and compassion, and we can stay together in unity. Despite the challenges families often go through, God is telling us that just as Christ's sacrifice offers redemption to humanity, families can experience redemption through fostering a deeper connection and reflecting God's grace. The bond of family transcends biological relationships. In Matthew 12:48–50 NIV, he says, "Who is my mother, and who are my brothers? …Whoever does the will of my Father in heaven is my brother and sister and mother." When it comes to family, look beyond biological relationships and prioritize spiritual bonds, because family is rooted in faith and values.

EMBRACING A NEW NORMAL AFTER LOSING OUR ROCK

Our life changed forever when my father died in a tragic accident. My siblings and I were still in elementary school, and his death devastated us. Every day I felt like there was this huge weight in my heart that wouldn't go away, yet life moved on, and I was still expected to show up as my best self. Faith in God and immense fortitude on the part of my mom kept the family going and helped me to deal with the loss. The teachers and most of the students showed me a lot of grace during the time I was struggling to come to terms with the loss of my father.

In the coming years, the financial status at home became more strained with our father gone. I had to take up work at a fast food restaurant when I was sixteen in order to help with some of the bills. I was so happy to help. My mother was also working extra hard; she took extra shifts at the hospital to a point where we hardly saw her because of how busy she would get. My job at the fast food restaurant took up much of my after-school hours. The money helped with family expenses and most things needed for school.

But I am no different from the millions of others working toward their dreams. Mine included some nightmares and some miracles. My journey, my ambition, my dreams are a testament to the shared hopes and struggles of many facing life's challenges. It is never easy to venture across oceans and continents just to seek a better life and future for yourself and your children. The journey is marred by both darkness and light; it takes a lot of perseverance, resilience, and unwavering determination to make it. Every time I look back at my life, I can't believe I made it this far, but my mother always taught me that God is with us.

The Lord says in Isaiah 41:10 and 13 NIV, "So do not fear, for I am with you; do not be dismayed, for I am your God. I will strengthen you and help you; I will uphold you with my righteous right hand. For I am the LORD, your God, who takes hold of your right hand and says to you, do not fear; I will help you."

These words carried me through. I was lucky enough to get admission to the University of South Florida where I followed in my sister Captain Julia's footsteps and enrolled in an Army ROTC college program, did basic training at Fort Lewis, Washington, and completed my medical training from the University of Arkansas where I served as the chief resident. Go Hogs! While in Arkansas, I started volunteer medical TV hosting for a show called *Family Health Today*. I'd do the show in between my ER shifts, sometimes still in scrubs, but at least I was able to teach and educate the community. It was fun, and it was my duty to serve my community.

My goal of becoming a doctor fulfilled, I moved to New York where I worked at a healthcare center on 42nd Street at Times

Square. This healthcare center felt like a battlefront war zone. Like a chaotic emergency room, it was nonstop trauma and drama.

REFLECTION

Life sometimes comes at you hard and fast; it hits you in such a way that you feel you no longer have the strength or the will to go on. God is reassuring us that He will always walk the journey with us, even in the face of loss and difficulties; we only have to trust in His divine strength. The Lord promises us His unwavering presence in our lives if we continue to dwell in His grace.

In Mathew 28:20 NIV, He says, "I am with you always, even to the end of this age."

As long as we obey the teachings of God, He will be with us always through every hardship or difficulty.

PRAYER

Almighty Father, thank you for always keeping us together, even when it feels like everything around us is falling apart. Thank you for your assurance that no matter how hard life gets, you will always walk the journey with us. All the blessings that come to us in life are through your divine will and grace. Thank you, Lord.

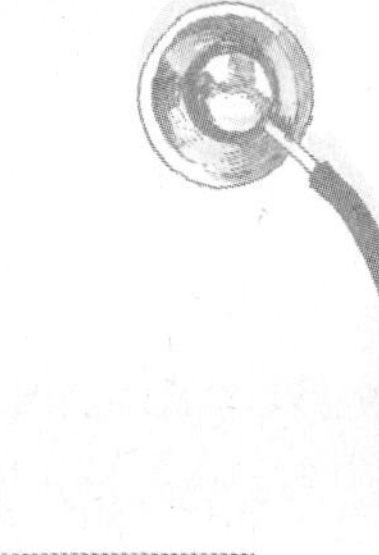

CHAPTER 4

MEDICAL TRAINING: DO NO HARM - FROM MEDICAL STUDENT TO CRISIS FIGHTER

During my medical training, I found myself on the front lines of two major health crises that imprinted upon me the critical role healthcare professionals play in times of urgent need.

The first was a severe flu outbreak, one that tragically claimed the lives of eighty thousand Americans. I was part of a team responsible for conducting mass flu clinics. People lined up, some looking visibly ill, waiting to be vaccinated or treated for flu. The queues were long, and the wait was agonizing for many. But, the weight of those eighty thousand lives loomed over us.

We worked diligently, one patient at a time, to curb the impact of the flu. Despite the exhaustion, the sense of urgency kept us going. Each shot we administered felt like a small but significant win in a larger battle. The flu shot can't stop you from catching the flu, but it can help reduce symptoms, and I've seen that firsthand with my patients.

THEN HURRICANE KATRINA HIT

However, during Hurricane Katrina, I faced one of the most challenging experiences of my medical training. I was in Chicago at the time, far from the eye of the storm, yet its impact reached us in a way we couldn't have imagined. Buses filled with hurricane survivors arrived at our makeshift emergency center, set up in a local gymnasium. These people had lost everything and arrived with a wide array of medical problems requiring immediate attention.

One case that stands out was a middle-aged African American man who came in with alarmingly high blood pressure—230 over 120 to be exact. He hadn't been able to take his medication because it was lost in the floodwaters back home. The situation was dire; he was on the verge of a stroke or heart attack. He was dizzy and short of breath. Our ambulances were already filled. In an unconventional but necessary move, we had to place two to three patients in a single ambulance to rush them to the hospital for immediate treatment.

Then, others had severe skin rashes and lesions from wading through the contaminated floodwaters. Their skin was raw, and their eyes were filled with pain and relief—pain from their physical condition and relief that they were finally getting medical help. Another case was a woman suffering from a severe asthma attack. She didn't have her inhaler and struggled with each breath she took. Her face showed her agony and a glimmer of hope as we administered a nebulizer treatment to relieve her symptoms. These were straightforward medical conditions, but one thousand at a single time made it tough. The key was triage.

Through these crises, I learned how crucial adaptability is in medical practice. Whether managing an unexpected influx of patients during a deadly flu season or providing emergency care after a natural disaster, flexibility, quick thinking, and a steadfast commitment to patient care were indispensable.

MY PERSPECTIVE CHANGED

Those experiences made me realize the full scope of my decision to pursue a medical career. It was not just about diagnosing illnesses or performing surgeries but also about being a beacon of hope and a source of relief during some of the most testing times in people's lives. There were instances when we had to bend the rules a bit, to ensure that people got the help they needed when they needed it the most.

As I look back at those demanding but formative years, I understand that they were not just part of my education but part of my becoming. The statistics—the eighty thousand lost to the flu and the countless affected by Hurricane Katrina—aren't just numbers. They were fathers, mothers, sons, and daughters. Behind each number was life, and the invaluable lessons I learned then continue to guide me in my medical practice today.

A healthcare professional's work is indeed never done in both calm and crisis. I carry this with me daily as I put on my white coat and step into the hospital, ready for whatever challenges come my way. Matthew 9:12 reminds me that the sick need our help.

FEAR'S GRIP NO MORE

I am no stranger to trauma; no doctors are. And I know fear very well, though less in myself than in the eyes of people I treated. But what I knew from my medical experience up to and through 2019 was different from what I was seeing in March 2020. All of my experience as a doctor up to that time boiled down to this: When catastrophe struck, it was a moment in time that came and went.

It left a broad sweep of suffering that had to be treated, but because the catastrophic event had passed away, we had a clear future with which to apply our medical remedies.

I remember volunteering in the aftermath of Hurricane Katrina in late August 2005. This was one of the great catastrophes laid upon the United States in modern times. Before Katrina, the most devastating natural disasters included the Great Chicago Fire of 1871, the Johnstown Flood of 1889, the San Francisco Earthquake in 1906, and Hurricane Andrew in Florida in 1992. Katrina was a Category 5 hurricane that pummeled New Orleans, Louisiana. It was the fourth most powerful storm to hit the mainland of the contiguous United States since recording storms began. The winds, rain, and storm surge were bad enough, but under this tremendous assault, the flood control system for New Orleans failed; 80 percent of the city's neighborhoods were flooded for weeks. Citizens were swept off their feet in floodwaters and swept away in their cars. Some scrambled to their roofs. If they were lucky, boats or helicopters soon took them away; if not, they just had to wait. The storm and its aftermath killed 1,800 people and caused $125 billion dollars in damage.

Mainly, during Katrina's aftermath, I worked in Chicago. New Orleans was a wreck, as were the rural communities for scores of miles around. So, the Federal Emergency Management Agency (FEMA) sent hundreds of victims on buses to Chicago. They were sheltered in large indoor areas such as gymnasiums. I worked in some of these where hundreds of traumatized survivors were sheltered with hardly anything but the clothes they were wearing when the hurricane had struck.

A few years later, I volunteered in Haiti after its horrible earthquake. It was a 7.0—exceptionally severe—whose center was at a town about fifteen miles southwest of the capital city Port-au-

Prince. Haiti has a population of about eleven million. Of these, it is thought one hundred thousand to three hundred thousand died when houses and buildings collapsed. About 250,000 homes and thirty thousand commercial buildings were severely damaged. In the capital, the National Palace, which serves as the president's residence, collapsed. For days and then weeks, people prodded through the rubble for the living and the dead. The injuries were horrible.

Add to this that Haiti is a very poor country—the poorest in the Western Hemisphere and one of the poorest in the world. The medical system is limited. And once you leave Port-au-Prince, you can't count on much, such as tolerable roads, reliable electricity, running water, and appropriate sewage disposal. Of course, all these were made even worse by the earthquake, so we had to work in exceptionally challenging conditions. Things were so bad in Haiti that in order to get there, we actually had to fly into the Dominican Republic. We'd hoped there would be a van there for us, but there was not. Someone found a beat-up van for us, and we bought it for about $3,000. We loaded it with as much equipment and supplies as we could. Then we drove up in the night into the mountains to cross into Haiti.

The roads were barely passable due to rockslides and mudslides that caused ruts and washouts. I recall at one point watching a road split open—tremors from the earthquake were still at work. In some parts of remote Haiti, you had to worry about robbers, kidnappers, and murderers. Where I eventually ended up working there was virtually nothing around—no resources at all: no light, no water. We stayed in huts. Sometimes we'd drive a couple of hours over barely passable roads to deliver what we could of health care.

I particularly remember caring for a newborn baby among the rubble. Normally when you deliver a baby, it's in a hospital. You have nurses, monitoring equipment, IVs at the ready, and trained nurses. I had none of these, except some towels brought by a villager, not even something with which to cut the cord. And it was scorching hot, probably around one hundred degrees. Someone had found a tent, and we were working inside, which made it seem all the hotter.

At least I had my stethoscope. When at last the baby was delivered, I could at least check the condition of her heart and lungs. Under the circumstances, the baby was in pretty good shape to begin life at such a time of natural disaster.

With no lights, it was pitch black at night. And the limited medical equipment and supplies we had had been barely suitable to the kinds of injuries and needs we were encountering. Fortunately, after a time, a team from Israel arrived in our region and then a team from the University of Miami. I arranged for the Arkansas hospitals where I had worked to provide fresh supplies.

We were all in danger, no doubt. It was a dangerous place. But the people were very grateful for what we could do for them. Here we could provide some help, some relief, especially when we went to the Ebenezer Orphanage in the village of Leogane filled with precious children.

HAITI: A JOURNEY OF COMPASSION AND RESILIENCE

So how did I end up in Haiti? After completing an extended shift at the hospital, I figured it was finally time to kick back and start my favorite unwinding routine—catching up on episodes of *M*A*S*H*, a show that beautifully explores the ideas of staying positive and strong when facing tough times.

So, there I was, sprawled on the couch, remote in hand, flipping through channels because I couldn't sleep after working overnight. But then, this one headline flashed on the screen: "Massive Quake Rocks Port-au-Prince, Haiti: Death Toll Soars, 356,769 Lives Lost."

Boom. Just like that, my mood went from a hundred to absolute zero. Shock, grief, and helplessness flooded in, drowning out any remnants of my earlier leisurely mood. I couldn't look away from those images—buildings crumbled, rescue teams slogging through the wreckage, and the faces of survivors etched with pain.

Amid this sad scene, my phone chimed, breaking the trance. My sister Jaclyn's text stared back at me, "Go help the babies!"

That's when this bolt of responsibility struck me—a deep, unshakable urge to take action. I placed the remote down and jumped into high gear.

Gathering up medical supplies from the hospitals I was connected with, pooling donations, and rallying my brother Danny and nephew Jon Paul, along with a pharmacist and a nurse who willingly jumped on board, became my mission.

Off we went to the Dominican Republic, meeting up with Pastor German from the church in Haiti. That drive, though—let's just say the roads weren't roads. It was more like a nerve-wracking, pitch-black roller coaster. My head practically had a competition with the Jeep's roof pole.

UNWAVERING COMPASSION

We set up camp and got to work. My local hospital where I worked donated lots of supplies for me to take with me. I was just a medical resident making $30,000 a year. I recall in the line at the airport, they wanted to charge me for all the supplies I was bringing with me. Everyone in the line started opening their wallets to help me pay for all the supplies to be shipped to Haiti, until the manager of the airline came out and waived all the hundreds, as it was for a good cause, humanity. Once on the ground, our first stop was the Ebenezer Orphanage, a haven for kids who were victims of the disaster. Then, it was on to Leogane village, where the struggles were raw—babies born on the streets, fractures, dehydration, infections, and young women seeking care. It was a chaotic mix of humanity's pain.

We dove into the chaos, working tirelessly until daylight faded away. And then, the darkness added another layer to the madness. The ground still trembled beneath us as we saw a city in ruins, its heartbeat silenced. Among the wreckage, I caught a snapshot of a child trying to bathe in a puddle—a reminder of the simple things we take for granted.

An unforgettable moment was when I had a banana, ate most of it, and tossed the last bit aside. As I turned unconsciously, I caught a child sifting through garbage for food then eating the remainder of the banana. It was like a punch in the gut, a stark reminder of what sheer poverty looks like—no food, shelter, or care. We couldn't turn away from this desperate plea.

I called my boss, Dr. Turner, back home in Fayetteville, telling him I wouldn't make my ER shift that weekend. Haiti held me tight. He understood and told me to be safe.

In time, the US military came to the rescue, their arrival a beacon of hope. Witnessing these teams lending a hand on a larger scale was beautiful. In an unexpected twist, an NFL team owner sent his private jet to pick us up after weeks of work and then being stranded. It was not easy to exit Haiti. Funny how help shows up in surprising forms.

I would have loved to go back again due to the extreme need to care for children, but with recent assassinations, crime, and kidnapping, I could not go. It's just too dangerous.

This journey brings to mind again Proverbs 3:5–6 NIV: "Trust in the Lord with all your heart and lean not on your own understanding; in all your ways submit to him, and he will make your paths straight." The path isn't clear, and the risks are real, but that unwavering trust keeps the fire burning within.

WHEN HEALTH COMES WITH A HEFTY PRICE TAG

Has one question changed your perspective on life? Perhaps it was, "Will you marry me?" or "Do you want this job?"

For me, working as a doctor in the ER a few years ago, that question came from Mark (not his real name), a critically ill patient I was attending to. He asked me, "How do I stop the transfer to another healthcare facility?"

I had encountered a patient whose predicament was as profound as it was tragic. A man caught in the cruel crossfire of two deadly ailments: a heart attack and blood cancer. His strength was ebbing away due to the relentless onslaught of his illnesses; his body weakened from the battle it was relentlessly waging.

His white blood cell (WBC) count was alarmingly high, hovering around one hundred thousand, a stark indicator of the severity of his condition. Yet, despite the grim prognosis, his concerns were not solely about his deteriorating health. Instead, they were rooted in something more profound, something that transcended his personal suffering—the financial burden that his treatment would impose on his family.

This man, frail and in the throes of pain, refused to be transferred to a hospital better equipped to manage his condition. The reason wasn't fear of the unknown or reluctance to leave familiar surroundings. No, his resistance was borne out of a fear far more gut-wrenching. He was terrified of the exorbitant cost of the treatment. He understood all too well that the price tag attached to his survival could plunge his family into crippling debt, a legacy he was unwilling to leave behind.

HEARTBREAKING DILEMMA

Mark's plight highlighted a heartbreaking dilemma that no one should ever face—choosing between life and financial ruin. It made me ponder—when did the value of a human life become so intricately linked with money? When did the will to survive come with a cost, literally and metaphorically?

The cruel irony of the situation was not lost on me. Here was a man facing the most challenging battle of his life, yet his primary worry was not about whether he would survive but about what his struggle for survival would cost his loved ones. His selflessness in the face of such adversity was both admirable and heartrending. He was willing to sacrifice his chance at life to ensure his family wouldn't have to bear the financial repercussions of his illness.

His story is not an isolated one. It represents a sad reality faced by countless individuals worldwide who are forced to weigh their health against their financial stability. More often than not, it's a choice they shouldn't have to make.

It led me to wonder—will there come a day when life is not contingent on money? When the cost of treatment won't instill fear in a patient's heart, overshadowing their fight for survival?

When will a person not have to worry about leaving a legacy of debt for their loved ones after their demise?

I yearn for a future where medical care is a right, not a privilege, where the pursuit of health does not come at the expense of financial security, where no one has to choose between their life and their livelihood, where access to affordable health care is a reality. Until then, we can only hope (as advised in 2 Corinthians 4:16–18), advocate, and strive for change.

After all, the true measure of any society can be seen in how it treats the most vulnerable members. In this regard, we still have a long way to go.

FIGHTING A CANCEROUS LUNG TUMOR

Sometimes, the most profound victories in medicine come after the most stubborn battles, not just against disease but against human nature itself. This was no more apparent than in the case of Mr. Thompson (not his real name), a patient who taught me that sometimes, pushing the boundaries of comfort is essential to save a life.

Mr. Thompson first walked into the clinic after experiencing persistent respiratory issues. A physician assistant (PA) had initially seen him and prescribed a Z-Pak, a common antibiotic for respiratory infections. However, three days later, he returned—more irritable and symptomatic than ever.

"Look, doc, the medication didn't work. I don't have time for this nonsense," Mr. Thompson grumbled, dismissing my suggestion for a chest X-ray (CXR).

For a moment, I considered respecting his wishes. After all, the autonomy of the patient is an important principle in medicine.

But then, I remembered the philosophy that I always aspired to follow: treat every patient as if they were family.

With a sense of paternal urgency, I chose to push the issue. "Mr. Thompson, I strongly recommend we get a chest X-ray. It's vital to understand what's happening in your lungs." We entered into a heated but respectful tug-of-war of words. He was difficult and resistant to the idea. Yet, I persisted, driven by an inexplicable sense that this was crucial.

CHEST X-RAY

Well, it's easy to feel defensive when a patient questions your judgment or expertise in the course of their treatment. However, I stayed calm, in control, and objective. Ephesians 4:32 highlights the importance of being kind and tenderhearted. So, I listened to Mr. Thompson's concerns and found a way to connect with him. Finally, he relented. He understood the importance of the chest X-ray.

"Alright, do your X-ray. But this better be worth it, and I want some strong cough medicine."

The X-ray images that popped up on my screen moments later left me stunned. There was an unmistakable mass. I felt a chill run down my spine as I called in a colleague for a second opinion. "Do you see what I see?" I asked, barely containing my incredulity.

"Yes, that's a mass," my colleague confirmed, mirroring my concern.

Subsequent tests proved our worst fears—it was cancerous. But there was a silver lining; we had caught it early enough for treatment to be feasible. Mr. Thompson started a rigorous course of therapy immediately.

The last chapter of this story unfolded on one New Year's Eve. I received an email that made all the struggles, the insistence, and the so-called "pushiness" worthwhile. It was from the patient, who had taken the time to hunt down my contact details. His email was short but filled with immense gratitude.

He was ringing in the New Year cancer-free, in remission, thanks to the early detection and subsequent treatment. I replied to his message with a heart full of joy and only three words, words that summed up my feelings and perhaps the divine intervention that had guided my actions: "Thank you, Jesus."

I learned that pushing someone a little can go a long way in pulling them back from the edge of death and despair. I learned to stay true to the values of medicine. Sometimes patient choices are the wrong ones, and it's my job to mend that or prevent it. I pray for the same outcome of remission for my precious young niece, who was diagnosed with leukemia. My brother, an attorney, was in court defending a case before the judge and the jury when I called him. It was tough having to break the news to my little brother that his daughter had cancer. It has been a roller coaster. There were times I thought God was about to take her home, but He did not. She is a fighter. I am grateful for every minute with her beaming smile. Leukemia patients who undergo chemotherapy have an extremely weak immune system, and fighting off a common cold could land them in the hospital or take their life. It is quite a humbling experience I wish upon no one.

TRIUMPH OVER GUILLAIN-BARRÉ: A YOUNG MAN'S JOURNEY AND A DOCTOR'S REVELATION

There was this young man, vibrant with life, who mysteriously began to experience an unsettling numbness and tingling sensation in his feet and legs, gradually creeping up to his thighs and stomach. He had been ill just a couple of weeks earlier with flu-like symptoms and a stomach bug, but these symptoms of numbness and tingling were distressingly unfamiliar. Seeking answers, he went to his personal doctor, but he did not improve, so he went to an emergency room, only to be told that it was just anxiety-induced hyperventilation and was told to breathe in a bag.

Days later, unsatisfied and still worried, he came to me. I was his third doctor visit, a fresh-faced physician stationed alone at Physicians' Specialty Hospital Sports Emergency Department in Fayetteville. As he narrated his ordeal, a mention of an upper respiratory tract infection and diarrhea from two to three weeks prior sent chills down my spine. This is the point I started getting a feeling about his ailment, and I had an idea of what this man was dealing with; could it be GBS? I ran some basic tests, blood work, and a CT scan. Guillain-Barré syndrome is a rare health condition that makes your body's own immune system cause damage to your nervous system. Each year, an estimated three thousand to six thousand people in the United States develop this disorder. Although anyone can develop this disorder, people older than fifty are at greater risk, according to the CDC. But unknown to most Americans, young people can also develop this health condition.

Alone and in need of specialized help, I reached out to a neurologist at another hospital and explained the man's illness. The doctor agreed to help my patient and accept him as a transfer for neurological care before the numbness, tingling, and weakness moved further to his diaphragm and lungs. Following thorough testing, my gut feeling was confirmed. The neurologist called me to tell me it was indeed Guillain-Barré syndrome. Time was of the essence! And the patient was immediately started on IV treatment to avoid paralysis and respiratory failure. You see, GBS can cause ascending paralysis, weakness that starts at the feet and works its way up to the diaphragm. If your diaphragm is paralyzed, you can't breathe. You die. Had I sent him home to "rest and stay hydrated," he would not have awakened the next morning.

The patient responded well to the treatment. This was evidence of the power of intuition and knowledge. At this point, I began to understand the medical profession better. It was like a new chapter in my life was opening.

It was as though all the textbooks I had poured over, all the lectures I had attended, and all the late-night study sessions had led me to this moment: the moment where I could make a difference, where I could save a life. And that victory was not just mine but also that of the young man who refused to ignore his body's signals and of the medical profession that equipped me with the knowledge to recognize and act. I attribute my ability to discern the disease to the intellect bestowed upon me, in that moment, by our Savior.

TO ALL DOCTORS OUT THERE...TO ALL THE HEALTHCARE PROVIDERS

Don't underestimate the good you can do for society, whether you are experienced or not. And always remember that every patient is a miracle waiting to happen. Jeremiah 33:6 reminds us about God's promise to heal us. It also reveals His promise to make us whole and bless us with an abundance of peace and security. God can heal someone through you.

Reflecting on this case, I am humbled and grateful. How did the experienced doctors before me miss it or dismiss this diagnosis as mere anxiety? And how did I, a novice, manage to identify it? I am grateful God was with me to take care of him.

I will never forget this case. It served as a reminder of the diversity of modern medicine. With thousands of diseases, every patient is a new challenge. But it's also a reminder of the responsibility physicians hold. And so, as I continue my work as a doctor, I am reminded to handle each patient carefully. Because sometimes, it's the "little ol' me,"' or the fresh-faced doctor, who makes all the difference.

AN INVISIBLE BATTLE: THE UNSEEN STRUGGLES OF MENTAL HEALTH

Deep within the labyrinth of modern society, often hidden from our sight, lie the foundations of homelessness, poverty, and drug addiction. At the heart of these struggles is an adversary, invisible yet powerful—mental illness. It's a battle that many fight in silence, their pleas for professional help often unheard. The path to the assistance they desperately need is often littered with challenges that seem endless, akin to scaling a mountain with no end in sight.

In a world where health insurance companies carefully design their policies like an intricate jigsaw puzzle, the importance of complete health care is overlooked. Psychiatric care, hearing aids, eyesight, and dental care—they all belong to the same body, the same person. Yet, they are treated as separate issues, leaving patients to struggle to access such services, especially mental healthcare services.

LACK OF ACCESS—THE LEADING CAUSE OF MENTAL HEALTH CRISIS

Federal laws require healthcare insurance providers to cover physical and mental health issues equally. However, deep disparities often exist between physical health insurance policies and policies that cover mental health. As a result, 42 percent of patients struggle to cover the high cost of mental healthcare services[1].

Even when you are insured through your parents, school, or job, treatments beyond medication can be costly. Recently, I had an experience that reminded me about the importance of accessibility and affordability of mental healthcare services.

One night at 42nd Street, a young mother of three walked in, cradling her baby. Her eyes were filled with despair so profound; it was palpable. She voiced her darkest fears, her urge to end her life and those of her innocent children. She told me she wanted to kill herself and her kids. As I listened, my heart pounded with a mix of relief and fear: relief that she had sought professional help and fear that she might flee before I could provide it.

I kept the door cracked open, maintaining a positive conversation with her—ensuring her safety and that of her children while awaiting psych care that was crucial. With every ounce of compassion and empathy, I spoke to her gently. I thanked her for her courage, praised her for seeking professional help, and reassured her that she had made the right choice. I reassured her that we were there to help her navigate this storm and ensure the safety of her beautiful family.

"Job 14:7–9 emphasizes the power of hope. Even when life's challenges knock you down, and you are probably feeling small, there's still hope. You can find strength in God and from your loved ones to support you and keep moving forward," I said to

---

1 National Council for Mental Wellbeing. "Study Reveals Lack of Access as Root Cause for Mental Health Crisis in America." The National Council for Mental Wellbeing. Published November 8, 2018. https://www.thenationalcouncil.org/news/lack-of-access-root-cause-mental-health-crisis-in-america/

her. I needed more help, but I couldn't leave her alone, unmonitored. Postpartum depression is not uncommon. It should be high on our internal alarm list as healthcare providers.

EXTERNAL FORCES THAT WORSEN MENTAL HEALTH

Reflecting on this case prompted me to think about other forces that worsen mental health. The pandemic lockdown further amplified the issue of mental health. The widespread lockdowns and unexpected disruptions in routines triggered more than just a wave of economic recession. About 41 percent of the United States adult population experienced high levels of psychological distress during the pandemic. And over a third of high school students reported mental health difficulties during the same period[2].

Social media addiction and suicidal ideation swelled like a tidal wave, sweeping countless individuals into its ruthless current. Alcohol and substance abuse, too, saw a steep rise. Research warns that adults who use social media excessively are three times more likely to suffer from anxiety and depression. This puts a significant percentage of the population at high risk for suicidal thoughts.[3]

---

2 Schaeffer, Katherine. "In CDC Survey, 37% of U.S. High School Students Report Regular Mental Health Struggles During COVID-19." Pew Research Center, April 25, 2022. https://www.pewresearch.org/short-reads/2022/04/25/in-cdc-survey-37-of-u-s-high-school-students-report-regular-mental-health-struggles-during-covid-19/.

3 University of Utah Health. "The Impact of Social Media on Teens' Mental Health." University of Utah Health, January 20, 2023. https://healthcare.utah.edu/healthfeed/2023/01/impact-of-social-media-teens-mental-health.

But in the face of these challenges, let us remember the resilience of the human spirit. Each one of us has the potential to be a beacon of hope, just like the young mother who sought help. Let's continue fighting for comprehensive health care, empathy, and understanding. Because at the end of the day, we're all part of the same body—humanity.

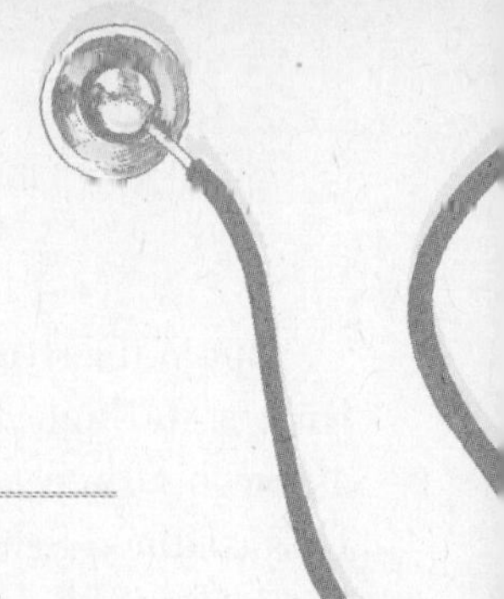

CHAPTER 5

Next Steps: Joplin Tornado

Another catastrophe I recall is when I worked after the Joplin, Missouri, tornado of May 2011. This tornado was an EF-5, the largest they get and far larger than the 2021 tornado that destroyed so much of Mayfield, Kentucky. The Joplin tornado, in fact, was the deadliest tornado in the United States since the 1940s. It killed 158 people and injured 1,500 more. I was working in Arkansas at the time. It was close by, so we went to help, as many needed medical attention, and the nearby hospital was blown out.

Most of us have never seen such a thing in real life—utter destruction everywhere. Houses and buildings were nothing but piles of rubble. All of the trees had been stripped of leaves, and the upper parts had been sheared away. It was unreal. I recall thinking that I must have been mistakenly put down on a movie set. Huge buildings like the Walmart Supercenter had been smashed to pieces and unroofed. The St. John's Regional Medical Center was destroyed. Large SUVs and cars lie flipped upside down on their roofs. So many people had been injured, dazed, depressed. Everything they had was gone, smashed or blown away. Naturally, we had to deal with the mental conditions as well as the medical ones.

But as horrific as these disasters were, everyone—and I include the medical staff—knew that the disasters themselves were a moment in time. Once the hurricane, earthquake, or tornado stopped, the skies cleared, and everyone knew the job was to mend as many of the survivors as rapidly as possible. For this, we had layers and layers of resources; we knew what the resources were, and we were confident that, properly applied, these resources would bring the community back together and most of the survivors back to reasonably good health.

This was definitely not the case with COVID-19.

A TALE OF RESILIENCE AND UNITY

When the Joplin tornado hit, I was living and working in northwest Arkansas. The sky turned a strange color that day, and you could feel something terrible was coming. Still, no one could have predicted the force of what hit us.

The local hospital was shattered, windows blown out, and walls caved in. Doctors and nurses were doing their best, but without electricity, it was like stepping back in time. Imagine a hospital where nothing works, where you can't even turn on a light or run a basic test. That's where we found ourselves.

The town was crushed. It looked like a scene from a movie, only this was real. No camera or special effects could capture the destruction, the heartbreak, and disbelief. Walmart, a place I had shopped at many times, imploded. Large SUVs were turned upside down like they were toys. Homes were flattened; years of memories and keepsakes vanished in seconds. You would look around and ask, "Is this really happening?"

COMING TOGETHER

But at that moment, something amazing happened. The people of the town, myself included, didn't let despair take over. Instead, we did what humans do best in times of crisis: we came together.

You wouldn't believe how fast people moved to help one another. Strangers helped pull people from the rubble. Neighbors who had never spoken were sharing food and water. Kids were helping elderly folks to safe spots. The spirit of the community was strong, stronger than the strongest winds of that tornado.

With no electricity and limited supplies, we became resourceful. We turned car headlights into emergency room lights. We used doors as makeshift stretchers. Everyone played a part. The local mechanic who could fix anything became a hero, making machines work against all odds. Teachers comforted children, telling them stories to keep them calm. Chefs cooked with whatever they could find, making sure everyone had something to eat.

And it didn't stop there. Help came pouring in from nearby towns and states. Trucks full of water, food, and medical supplies arrived. Doctors and nurses from other hospitals came to lend a hand. Even people who had lost everything were finding ways to help. A woman whose house was destroyed set up a small stand to hand out free iced tea and water.

A group of kids organized a toy drive for those who had lost their belongings. A local musician played songs to lift people's spirits. You felt like crying, but you also felt like cheering. The town faced tough days, weeks, and months ahead. Rebuilding lives was not easy, but they did it step by step, day by day. And they did it together. The tornado took their homes and belongings, but it didn't take their spirit.

Years have passed, but the memories remain vivid. The hospital has been rebuilt, this time stronger and more resilient. The town, too, has come back to life, and you can see signs of new beginnings everywhere you look. Even the people seem to stand a little taller, knowing that they faced the worst and came out stronger on the other side.

Whenever I think back to that time, I don't just remember the destruction. I remember the heroes—everyday people who showed the best of humanity. I remember the kindness, the courage, the love that poured forth from the heart of a broken community. And I realized, if you could get through that, you can get through anything.

And so, even when the skies turn dark, and life throws its worst at us, we know we'll be okay. Because we're not just a town; we're a community, a family—1 John 4:12 emphasizes this unity. And when you have that, you can weather any storm.

THE DAY A PARKING LOT BECAME A LIFESAVER

I worked in the emergency room in a small rural town called Eureka Springs in Arkansas. I was still learning as a second-year medical resident. This wasn't a big city hospital but a small, three-bed ER. We faced unique challenges there—especially the shortage of doctors. I was one of the few trained right there in Arkansas, trying to give back to the place I called home.

Then came a day I will never forget—a test of my skills, patience, and hope.

A young boy, not older than seven, had an accident at a local park. He flew fifteen feet off a swing and slammed his head on the concrete. When he came into the ER, I saw his condition, stabilized him, and knew he needed specialized care—care we couldn't provide. So, I called for a medical helicopter to take him to a children's trauma center after acceptance from the on-call neurosurgeon.

We prepared him for the journey, ensuring he was stable. His parents, eyes filled with worry, watched as we wheeled him out to the helicopter. But then, in a twist of fate, the stretcher hit the helicopter's windshield frame and cracked it. The pilot checked the damage and shook his head. "We can't fly like this. It's too dangerous."

My heart sank. Every second mattered for this young boy; now, we had no time to spare. He could at any minute seize, have internal bleeding, or go unconscious due to internal bleeding and swelling in his brain. I didn't have a cranial drill to drill a burr hole in his skull to decompress his brain from the pressure of swelling and bleeding. Inspired, I thought about the local McDonald's parking lot—large enough for a helicopter to land and not too far from the hospital. We didn't have a moment to lose.

"We'll use the McDonald's parking lot," I told the team. "Get another chopper here, now!"

The paramedics rushed the boy back into the ER while we waited for the second helicopter. His mom and dad followed, their faces etched with lines of fear and hope. The waiting was the most challenging part, but the roar of helicopter blades finally filled the air.

SAVING A LIFE

We moved quickly. As we wheeled him out again, this time to the McDonald's parking lot, the whole team felt the weight of the situation. This was it. The helicopter touched down, and we transferred him carefully, ensuring no more mistakes.

As the helicopter lifted into the sky, I felt relief and hope. The young boy was going to get the care he desperately needed. His parents thanked us, their eyes speaking what words could not convey.

Days later, we got the news. The boy had made it through neurosurgery and was on his way to recovery. A collective sigh of relief spread through the ER. We knew we had made a difference, even if it was just for one young boy in a small town in Arkansas.

That day taught me important lessons. It showed me that medicine is not just about what you learn from textbooks; it's about thinking on your feet and using what you have. It's about a community coming together, from the helicopter pilots to the staff at McDonald's who cleared the parking lot in a heartbeat.

But most of all, it taught me about hope—the hope in the eyes of a young boy's parents, the hope of a community for better health care, and the hope in myself to be the best doctor I can be right there where I started, in Arkansas.

So, when people ask me why I chose to stay and work in a place with a shortage of doctors, I think of that young boy and that fateful day. Then I smile and say, "Because this is home, and home is where you make a difference." 1 Peter 4:10 NIV reminds us to use our gifts to help others.

TURNING DESPAIR INTO HOPE DURING THE UKRAINE CRISIS

In a world where the news brought me heartache day after day, I knew I had to act. I could no longer be just a spectator to the suffering of the Ukrainian people. I saw a child lost forever on a hospital stretcher as the medics performed compressions and gave her epinephrine to start her heart, and something inside me screamed, "Enough!" In the heart of Ukraine, amid the echoes of conflict, I found myself on a medical mission like no other before. The war-torn landscape served as a backdrop for my journey where courage and faith were tested in the crucible of adversity.

Gathering supplies and medical kits, I shared my decision with family and friends. I was going to Ukraine to provide medical care for the wounded. My brother Danny, who had been with me on a medical mission to Haiti, offered to go with me. My nephew Jon Paul and a few other colleagues also joined our team.

We landed in Poland, near the Ukraine border, intending to set up a medical camp there. But soon, I got a call. The plea was desperate: "We need you inside Ukraine." The decision weighed heavily on me. I prayed, seeking some guidance, and it became clear. I had to go. I left Danny and the team at the border to care for the refugees there while I ventured into the unknown.

Once in Ukraine, we took shelter underground beneath a shopping plaza. I was part of a disaster assist relief team (DART). The air was heavy with the sound of sirens and the smell of smoke. Despite the chaos, the indomitable spirit of those in need who were unjustly attacked fueled my determination where each day became a testament to the human spirit's ability to persevere. But in the midst of it all, I began to work. I worked in a makeshift clinic at the bottom of the railway station in L'viv. Here, trains carried the wounded, the sick, and the hopeless from places like Kiev and Kherson. And there, I met them with everything I had: medicine, skill, and love.

THE HOUR OF NEED

Little children with missing fingers, people with burned legs, those suffering from heart attacks, asthma attacks, pneumonia, one lady with a severely deformed wrist fracture that needed surgery, but she only wanted pain killers and then to continue fleeing out of Ukraine to reach safety—my days became a blur of faces and diagnoses. Yet, each face reminded me of why I was there—to bring some relief, some hope, some prayer in their hour of need. One woman, a poet, told me how difficult it was trying to flee on the train out of Ukraine. I asked why. She told me, with tears rolling down her face, their train was being shot at by Russians. I told her, "You are safe now; no one can hurt you," and I hugged her.

In one remarkable moment, a train conductor sprinted toward me as I was working in a tent at the L'viv railway in Ukraine. A woman had collapsed on one of the trains. Without a second thought, I ran up the stairs, leaped across the tracks, and rushed to her. With each step, I carried the collective support of all those who had sent me on this mission, all those who had said, "Go. Help them."

One elderly man was vomiting, severely dehydrated and weak. I placed an IV to hydrate him and found some old Zofran nausea medicine in my bag. It helped tremendously, but then one fateful day, the wail of alarm sirens went off, which meant we had to rush underground to seek safety from the bombings and incoming attacks. We had to carry our sick and injured patients with us underground. I am strong, I do push-ups every morning, but it was tough carrying other large humans. Teamwork made it easier. The world outside transformed into a chaotic symphony of distant explosions. My adrenaline was pumping, my heart pounding as I guided patients through the labyrinthine corridors underneath the railway. The pressure of my duty and obligations weighed heavily upon me, literally. The underground shelter beckoned as a sanctuary against impending danger. Walking down dimly lit passages felt like a surreal odyssey. The atmosphere thick with tension intensified the sense of purpose that motivated us. The unwavering commitment to take care of each other and the bonds forged in adversity were the defining narrative of that day I'll never forget. In the shelter's dim light, I continued to provide medical care, my hands steady despite the palpable tension—where did this unyielding will to serve, even in the shadows of war, come from? It must be my mom. My dear friend Dr. Olsen said to me, "Dr. J, are you brave or crazy?"

I answered, "Probably both, eighty/twenty."

It was very cold and dark in the underground tunnel, but at least we were safe for the time being. At the end of my shift, our incredibly helpful translator and driver, Denis, would drive us back to the shopping center where we slept underground in tents. I remember hearing odd noises, wondering what those noises were. I kept asking, "What is that noise?" but nobody answered me. Finally, a nurse told me they were bombs going off. They didn't want to tell me because they didn't want me to get scared. I couldn't sleep that night. I didn't know how we would get home alive. It was freezing cold underground. I only worried about who would take care of my widowed mom if something happened to me. Otherwise, I was not afraid to die, because I knew I was serving God.

In those intense days and nights, I often thought about what had brought me there. I was reminded of a greater purpose, a divine calling to serve not just myself but others. God puts us on Earth for a reason, and in those challenging moments, I felt I was living mine. Psalm 46:1 reminds us of God's promise to strengthen us, even in a time of need.

Back at the Poland-Ukraine border, Przemyśl, Danny and the team were also working tirelessly. They had set up a medical camp that became a beacon of hope for thousands of Ukrainian families fleeing the bombing and the destruction of their homes. Though separated by miles, our united purpose transcended the distance.

Eventually, I returned to my home country, but a piece of my heart stayed in Ukraine. And a piece of Ukraine came back with me—captured in videos of sirens and photos of smoky skies imprinted on my soul forever.

Sometimes, when the world presents us with overwhelming darkness, we find our true light. I did. And it taught me that when faced with the choice between being a spectator or a healer, always choose to heal. It's in that choice that we find our true purpose, guided by a higher power and driven by an unwavering love for humanity.

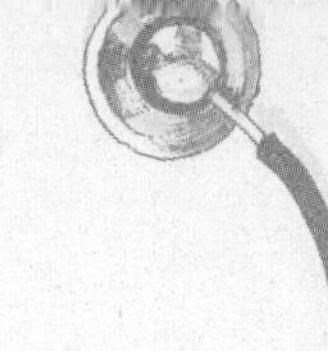

CHAPTER 6

Tenderness, Clarity, Compassion

The trauma of her past is still palpable. Several years later, Jane (not her real name) agreed to speak to me about her situation for the first time. I cannot disclose her name to protect her identity. To this day, she is still terrified.

Amid the glaring lights of the city, there's a street known to many but spoken about by few—57th Street. Here, the shadows hold stories—ones of pain, survival, and, often, hope. Jane's is one such story. Young and incredibly beautiful, Jane was more than what met the eye. The world saw her as a prostitute, but behind those captivating eyes lay a tale of adversity and courage.

One evening, Jane came in visibly distressed in a medical facility just a few blocks down 57th Street. Accompanied by a man—her "date"—she had severe genital ulcers, a health issue that had her anxious. She seemed afraid of something more than the infection.

She was frantic as to how she would pleasure her date with this infection; I started her on meds and told her to avoid sexual activity at this time. She asked me if she could "do oral," as she was so desperate to serve and satisfy him to be paid. But I could sense her despair and silent "cry for help."

THERE'S A CHANCE SHE WAS FORCED INTO PROSTITUTION

As a healthcare provider, I was trained to attend to the ailment, but Jane's genuine despair required more than just medical treatment. I asked her companion to step out for doctor-patient privacy. The man was hesitant initially, but after a short back-and-forth, he agreed to step out.

As soon as the door clicked shut, Jane's strong façade crumbled. Tears streamed down her face. Behind being a prostitute, her circumstances, and her choices, she was just a young woman scared for her health and future. She whispered through her tears about the desperation of the moment, the urgency to satisfy her client so she could be paid.

As I listened, a chilling thought crept into my mind. Could she have been a victim of trafficking at a tender age? But before I could ask, Jane broke down.

"This isn't the future I envisioned. I was abused from a young age, and now I have to live in a violent environment to make a living. I feel safe when I'm with Joe [the man she walked in with]. But I still have to service another five or more men a day to make a living. There's always a chance they could turn violent...."

A SHRED OF HOPE FOR HER

I gently intervened as she narrated her story and raised more questions about her current predicament. I told Jane that there was a life full of opportunities and different paths beyond her present moment and her immediate needs. I spoke of faith, seeking God, praying, and finding strength.

I encouraged her to believe in herself, to understand that she was more than her job and that the choices she made today could reshape her tomorrow. I stood up, placed my hand on her shoulder, and said, "Jane, God hears your cry of pain. He will always be your foundation when everything else seems to fall apart. When you get home, read Psalm 40:1–3, and you will find strength in faith."

Psalm 40:1–3 NIV says, "I waited patiently for the LORD; he turned to me and heard my cry. He lifted me out of the slimy pit, out of the mud and mire; he set my feet on a rock and gave me a firm place to stand."

Jane looked up, her tear-streaked face glistening under the sterile white lights. I saw a glimmer in her eyes—a spark of hope, perhaps for the first time in a while.

As she walked out with her "date," thoughts streamed through my mind. This girl from 57th Street can be transformed and take control of her narrative. Though still unfolding, her journey can become a testament to the indomitable human spirit and the transformative power of hope and faith in God. And I would feel blessed to have played a part in her story of redemption. While I do not know what happened to Jane, I do hope that she found strength to bring about positive change in her life and I continue to pray for her.

Prostitution and all related activities—including maintaining brothels and pimping—fuel the growth of modern-day human trafficking and slavery. They often provide a façade behind which human traffickers and pimps practice sexual exploitation. Most women and young girls don't want to be there. While few choose it, most are desperate to leave it.

I witnessed sexual abuse in my immigrant non-English-speaking patients. Many were young teenage girls. Sadly, I had one young Hispanic teenager who didn't speak English; she had been in New York for a few weeks, staying at a local shelter, and was raped by another illegal immigrant in the shelter. She broke down and cried, her mother cried, and I began to tear up, heartbroken for what she had endured due to our loss of control at our southern border.

This reminds me of the young women I cared for at the Poland-Ukraine border who were raped and assaulted by Russian soldiers. They were pregnant, they had pelvic inflammatory disease, and they were scared, in pain and alone. I am grateful to God I was able to help them heal. I stayed in a tent and used a wood oven to stay warm—it was hard to keep the wood on fire. I learned how to chop my own wood out there to stay warm.

CHAPTER 7

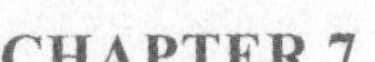

Mysterious Epidemic Strikes Wuhan

I vividly recall that in December of 2019, the medical community began to see reports of a new virus that was sickening the people of Wuhan, China. Wuhan is the capital city of Hubei Province, which is west of Shanghai, in the middle of the country. It has eleven million inhabitants and is the largest city in central China, slightly larger than New York City with nine million people. It is important to note that Wuhan is also the location of the Wuhan Institute of Virology (WIV), a laboratory created in the 1950s that is administered by the Chinese Academy of Sciences, which in turn reports to the nation's communist government. The WIV was the first in China to operate as a biosafety level 4 (BSL-4) laboratory, the highest level of biosafety precautions. It has close associations with laboratories in other countries, including the United States. This vital information was not known by many and thus an extremely significant fact that gave birth to the plague that hit our country.

The WIV is particularly noted for its research into severe acute respiratory syndrome (SARS) viruses, and especially coronaviruses, which make up a large family of viruses that cause infections in the nose, sinuses, and throats of both mammals—including, of course, humans—and birds. The "common cold" can be caused by several kinds of viruses—rhinoviruses, adenoviruses, enteroviruses...and coronaviruses.

Coronaviruses come in different forms, and they can mutate quickly. They are the viruses responsible for the SARS breakout of 2003 originating in China and spreading to four other countries.

When we began to see reports of a new variant of coronavirus in Wuhan and of Wuhan residents suffering from respiratory infections, we immediately had to pay attention.

As a doctor, I can tell you that human disease has many sources, but chief among them are bacteria and viruses. Bacteria are so small that it was not until the nineteenth century and the use of microscopes that medical researchers understood some types of these very small, single-cell organisms attack cells in the human body and cause disease. Typically, bacteria are one-half to five microns large. By comparison, a human hair measures about seventy-five microns wide. In the twentieth century, medical researchers learned how to create antibiotic medicines that kill many types of harmful bacteria, ones, for example, that can cause cholera, tuberculosis, and typhoid fever.

Once nineteenth-century medicine discovered that some bacteria caused disease, doctors and scientists believed for a time that bacteria caused all diseases. So, medical researchers were dismayed when they could find no bacteria causing such illnesses as measles, mumps, polio, and influenza. That's because these diseases, including colds, are caused by viruses—microbes so small that the microscopes of the medical researchers did not detect them. This is because viruses are about one hundred times smaller than bacteria.

Viruses, in fact, can easily travel in water droplets expelled from people when they cough or sneeze, and even in droplets that are smaller than those coughed or sneezed, and that drift around for a long time in the currents of the air. People inhale these droplets and then the viruses attack cells in their respiratory system. This is why viral diseases are so contagious. The other means of widespread contagion is when people with a virus get the virus on their fingers when they touch their mouth, nose, or eyes and then transfer the viruses on their fingers to doorknobs or other objects they touch. The viruses, like flu, are once again transferred to the fingers of uninfected people who admit the virus into their bodies when they use their fingers to touch their mouth, nose, or eyes. Transmission can happen in mere seconds in this manner—not a big deal when we're talking about the common cold but something else entirely when we're dealing with a virus of unknown origin and with potentially devastating consequences. "Brace for Impact" was on every healthcare worker's mind.

We were very concerned. We were especially worried when we saw the video reports from Wuhan. We could see that the laboratory and health workers there were wearing space suit-like gear, the kind we had not seen much of since the Ebola outbreak of 2014–2016. (The Ebola virus can kill 50 percent of the people it infects.) We in the United States were alarmed at what we were seeing and hearing: eleven million people forced to stay home was a bad sign.

The Chinese government quarantined the entire city of Wuhan. We understood that if the Institute of Virology thought enough of this newly discovered virus to require full precautionary gear—PPE—as well as a quarantine of the city, then officials there must suspect both that the virus could cause serious disease and that it was going to be difficult to contain. The first confirmed death of a Wuhan resident owing to the new illness was announced in early January. Still, on account of what looked like a very credible effort by the local Wuhan and Chinese governments to contain the virus, many in the United States were not worried; they believed the disease wasn't going to hit them because of the measures in place in Wuhan meant to confine the disease to central China. That was far from the truth.

The easy transmission of the disease overwhelmed the containment efforts of the Chinese. I recall discussing this with Neil Cavuto on air; his suspicion was right on target early on in the pandemic that the CCP was hiding something. Almost a month after the first Wuhan virus death, that is, near the end of January, the virus arrived in the United States when a person in Washington State was diagnosed with it. Italy soon became an infection hot spot. At the end of January, the World Health Organization (WHO) announced a "Public Health Emergency of International Concern." Earlier in the month, on January 5, 2020, the WHO announced that "of the 44 cases reported, 11 are severely ill, while the remaining 33 patients are in stable condition. According to media reports, the concerned market in Wuhan was closed on 1 January 2020 for environmental sanitation and disinfection." At the time, the WHO did not recommend "any specific measures for travelers."

But the statements became more dire by the day. In February, the International Committee on Taxonomy of Viruses named this new virus SARS-CoV-2. It also gave a name to the disease the virus caused—COVID-19, the "19" referring to 2019, the year the disease was discovered. In early March, the virus was spreading in Europe and the United States. On March 11, the WHO declared a worldwide pandemic. The director-general's opening remarks were sobering, revealing to a panicked world that over 118,000 cases had already been identified in 114 countries, with 4,291 people already dead. "We have never before seen a pandemic sparked by a coronavirus," Tedros Adhanom Ghebreyesus said. "This is the first pandemic caused by a coronavirus. And we have never before seen a pandemic that can be controlled, at the same time."

We braced ourselves. But we could not be sure what was going to happen. In Italy, COVID-19 patients were dying at a disturbingly high rate. Would that happen in the United States? In New York City? Fear and panic spread quickly.

I am sure we had COVID cases earlier in the year of 2020, but I did not have swabs to test them. I saw my first confirmed COVID patient in March 2020. Little did we know that that mother, that patient, was only the first of waves that would come one after another crashing on our shores.

Wave after wave after wave.

Trying to be hopeful, we didn't yet know of the future deluge of infected patients that would soon overwhelm our center.

The patients kept coming. Our spirits began to waver, especially as the kinds of patients coming through our doors weren't the typical ones with preexisting medical conditions or suffering a sudden disease. Healthy people were suddenly unable to breathe. Very unusual, nonstandard illnesses with undiagnosable symptoms were pouring in. I remember a patient who came in with a high fever. It was the first time I put on an N95 mask with a head to toe PPE gown and face shield. I remember hoping and praying his flu swab would come back positive and it did. I felt relieved. I thought he was out of the woods but looking back, it was possible to have both the flu and COVID at the same time—that could have been deadly.

I will never forget my first serious COVID patient: a sixty-year-old man brought in by his wife who nearly collapsed in my arms. He was tall and felt very weak. He had been sick for about ten days already. His oxygen level was hovering in the seventies. Normal oxygen is in the nineties. We slipped on an oxygen mask, set the valve to high flow, and whisked him off to be admitted to the hospital because the oxygen tank I had was running out of oxygen. I had confidence he would recover. I suspected COVID-19, but I didn't have any swabs left to test him. His wife tested positive. I figured I would go by process of elimination. His flu was negative, his chest X-ray showed a snowy whiteout pattern typical of COVID, and his vitals were so bad that he needed to be hospitalized immediately. As he was rolled away on a stretcher, he looked at me and nodded, and I smiled back, gave him a thumbs up. I thought he'd be all right since I got his oxygen level back up to normal, he perked up, and looked okay. I called to check on him a few days later, but there was no answer. I called again the next day; his wife answered the phone crying. I was shocked to learn he had died that night he was admitted. Even the ventilator at the hospital couldn't save him. He did have a history of A-fib, a heart disease. I often wondered had he not been intubated if he would have survived. This reminded me to check on my friend Maria, who only had one lung. I was so worried about her, but I was also so overwhelmed with patients. In the back of my head, I kept saying, call her, check on her, call her…then before I had the chance to, I saw one day she had passed from COVID. I was so saddened.

That's when the growing fear set in for my staff. I had a young nineteen-year-old female with a history of mild asthma complain she couldn't breathe. Her anxiety and shortness of breath were palpable. This respiratory disease was a killer. Trucks were used as morgues as people were dying left and right at the start of the pandemic. After seeing the outbreak in Italy, what would stop it from coming to the United States? We knew two things: one, that COVID had come to New York City, and the first strain was killing people not otherwise compromised with other problems or morbidities ("morbidities" is the medical term for diabetes, heart disease, immune deficiencies, and the like); and two, that as people who worked all day with sick patients, we ourselves could contract the disease, and it could kill us. And not just that—we could innocently take it home to our families, where it would kill them, too, or just make them sick, or in the case of children, have no symptoms at all.

I couldn't stop thinking about my widowed mom living in Tennessee. I missed her terribly, and I wished I could be surrounded by my family during this trying and difficult period. But concern of losing loved ones was exacerbated because I was caring for COVID patients all day long, seeing them sick and dying while trying to help them; I called Mother any chance I got just to check up on her. One of the biggest challenges that the pandemic brought was loneliness and ostracization from family, friends, and loved ones. People had to take unprecedented isolation and distancing measures in order to protect themselves and their loved ones from contracting the virus. Some of the measures the government put in place to reduce the spread of the virus were lockdowns, quarantines, and social restrictions. This meant that many people could not be with loved ones or travel to comfort and see them. This created a big disconnect for many. There were no face-to-face meetings, so many people had to shift to remote work and online communications only. In the face of fear, worry, and even anxiety, this only amplified feelings of loneliness and vulnerability for many individuals. It was indeed a difficult period. We should have stayed focused on the high-risk population and not shut down the nation. The lockdowns and social restrictions did not work. I know this firsthand working on the front lines of COVID.

PRAYER

Almighty and ever-loving Father, you are God above all adversities and epidemics. We call upon your name that you may protect us, cover us with your precious blood that was shed in Calvary, oh Father, that no harm may come to us, that sicknesses and viruses may never be our potion. May you protect our families and always keep us together in your love. Amen.

REFLECTION

The onset of this pandemic can be seen as a great time for spiritual contemplation and reflection on our paths as Christians. When you face difficult times, it is always a good opportunity to slow down and reconnect with your maker. Turn to your faith for solace and find guidance through the word of God. It is easy to become disillusioned and sad during hard times, so these are the times you need God more. Take the opportunity when everything has slowed down in the world to strengthen your relationship with God.

The pandemic also helped us to appreciate more the importance of community. Sometimes you take love for our neighbors, friends, and even family for granted. But with a pandemic, it was obvious that sometimes in the blink of an eye we can lose some of our most cherished connections with people. People die and sometimes you just can't be with them even though you want to. So be loving and compassionate towards one another, because you never know when you will need someone most, yet you can't be with them. I love that many people found innovative ways to support and reach out to one another amid the restrictions and distancing measures. After all, the greatest commandment of all is love. God says in 1 Peter 4:8 NKJV, "Above all, keep loving one another earnestly, since love covers a multitude of sins," and in John 15:12 NIV, "My command is this: Love each other as I have loved you."

WAVES OF COVID-19

I've described COVID as waves breaking on a beach. One comes and you try as best you can to deal with it. And then another comes, and you deal with that. And then another comes and another and another. We had no idea when these waves would stop, how large they would become, when we could catch our breath, or when we could see that "the end was in sight." We saw people dying, some young, healthy, some doctors, some nurses.

COVID was indeed different. We were not working in a gymnasium with people lined up for treatment. We were not working in a sparsely populated area of a Caribbean country. We were not in a small city where, though huge sections were rubble, the number of people needing medical care was known and decreasing by the day.

Instead, in New York City, we were in the middle of the largest as well as the most densely populated city in the nation. Above and around our healthcare center were buildings a thousand feet high holding the offices or living spaces of millions of people. Outside our healthcare center walked thousands of people each day, hundreds in a single hour, and all of whom appeared rather healthy. But some of them might be—in fact, even in January, most certainly were—infected with the SARS-CoV-2 virus that was highly contagious.

We could not be sure what the next months would do to us. We well understood that we could not have regular New Yorkers wear the head-to-toe PPE used in the Wuhan Institute of Virology. We knew we could not stop New Yorkers from talking, turning doorknobs, pushing elevator buttons, taking shopping bags from retail clerks, or coughing and sneezing in crowded subway cars. We silently counted the number of beds in the city's hospitals and the number of beds in the hospital intensive care wards compared to the number of inhabitants—eleven million—in the city's five boroughs. We thought of hundreds of thousands of residents over sixty-five or who suffered from diabetes, heart or lung problems, that is, the people the most vulnerable to a virus that attacked the lungs and shut down breathing.

We wondered if we should begin to imagine this huge city, so dependent on human contact, meetings, and gatherings of all sorts, becoming a metropolis of millions of people afraid of talking to one another or of even approaching one another, a city of empty offices, empty theaters, and empty schools, of thousands lined up at hospital doors begging to be let in, and of coffins stacking up at cemeteries for want of enough gravediggers to keep up with the need to bury them.

We wondered. We tried to repress these thoughts. But we really didn't know. We couldn't be sure what the future was going to hurl at us.

We went to work at our healthcare center each day, and we hoped—we hoped fewer rather than more people would show up with breathing problems.

It was not to be.

I began thinking about my own family and how I might keep them safe.

PRAYER

Dear Lord, you are our refuge in times of sorrow, adversity, and uncertainty; we have nowhere else to seek solace and strength. That is why we run to you, we pray for all the people who have been affected by COVID-19, we pray for all the lives that have been lost and for all the families that are grieving their loved ones. We pray for the healthcare workers and all the frontline workers who worked tirelessly to help those affected; protect them and give them the resilience to continue serving your people selflessly. May we find strength in your grace to overcome all the challenges of COVID. Amen.

REFLECTION

If anything, COVID-19 was a stark reminder of the fragility of human life and existence; life can change without warning. So, as a Christian, how prepared are you when the changes come? How did the epidemic affect your faith? Did your belief grow stronger, or did it wane under the pressure of the epidemic?

Times like these compel us to reflect on the fundamental truths of our beliefs as Christians. Do your beliefs give you any solace? If they do not, then it is time to reassess your beliefs. The word of God and the truth of Christ offer comfort, solace, and guidance to all those who seek them. The scripture has words of encouragement to all of us no matter what circumstance you're facing in life. I remember every time I called my mom to check up on her, she was always very hopeful. She always spoke words of encouragement to me because most of her time in lockdown was spent caring for her grandkids and reading the Bible. Thanks, Mom.

Her attitude reminded me of God's promise in Isaiah 40:31 KJV that "they who wait for the Lord shall renew their strength; they shall mount up with wings like eagles; they shall run and not be weary; they shall walk and not faint."

This is your reminder to wait on the Lord, for those who wait on the Lord never grow weary.

NAVIGATING THE STORM: UNPRECEDENTED UNCERTAINTY GRIPS THE WORLD

> As we continue to provide essential updates and encourage people to act upon the facts on coronavirus instead of the hype, I have officially done a declaration of emergency which gives us certain powers to help local health departments that are very stressed. As the local health departments continue to monitor and quarantine people, we have a more expedited purchasing protocol to get them all the tools they need to contain the virus spread.
>
> —Governor Andrew Cuomo declaring a state of emergency in New York, March 7, 2020

A palpable sense of concern gripped the city's residents in the wake of Andrew Cuomo's declaration of a state of emergency. The once bustling streets of New York slowly transformed into quiet and deserted streets as news of the virus spread. The city that never sleeps had been forced into a slumber; once packed with commuters, subway platforms now bore an eerie sense of emptiness as the government advised travelers against using public transportation. The ones who still dared to use the public transportation system showed up in face masks and gloves and kept a considerable distance from one another. Remote work became the new normal as more companies and businesses adjusted to telecommunications to reduce face-to-face meetings. In response to the crisis, the government took swift measures to curb the spread of the virus; they put up health checkpoints at significant intersections where medical professionals distributed masks and checked to see if anyone had the virus.

But at first, there was a surge of activity, with many rushing to stock up on essential things they would need while on lockdown. Grocery store lines snaked around corners while local shops had an insane number of customers who left many empty shelves behind them. The government even had to call on people to only take enough for themselves and leave some for other people and families. Many families that did not rush to the shops quickly missed many essentials, which isn't what God teaches us in His word. Taking more than you need at the expense of other families goes against Christian teachings and the word of God. It shows a lack of consideration, empathy, and compassion for the well-being of others, and these are values that have been highlighted and emphasized in the Bible.

Philippians 2:4 NKJV says, "Let each of you look out not only for his own interests, but also for the interests of other."

The Bible further underscores the importance of treating others as you would like them to treat you. Hoarding essential supplies and leaving others in need reflects a failure to love our neighbors as ourselves. The scripture says in Matthew 22:39 NIV, "And the second is like it: 'Love your neighbor as yourself.'"

It is understandable that there was a high sense of uncertainty, as nobody knew how long they would have to stay in isolation, but during times like this, our Christian values are tested the most. I can't help but laud the people whose community spirit flourished during this period. Many New Yorkers rallied together by organizing food drives for the vulnerable population. They fed the homeless and sent food, clothing, and other essential goods to homeless shelters. This is what God teaches us to do; for in 1 John 3:17–18 NIV, we are told, "If anyone has material possessions and sees a brother or sister in need but has no pity on them, how can the love of God be in that person? Dear children, let us not love with words or speech but with actions and in truth."

James 2:15–16 NIV further highlights the importance of taking concrete actions to help those in need rather than just preaching it. It says, "Suppose a brother or a sister is without clothes and daily food. If one of you says to them, 'Go in peace; keep warm and well fed,' but does nothing about their physical needs, what good is it?"

Many people also showed a great appreciation for healthcare workers by sewing masks for them, and there was also the famed "cheers for carers," a move that was meant to appreciate healthcare workers. Every night at 7 p.m., neighbors of healthcare workers would stand in their balconies or driveways and give a round of applause to healthcare workers and first responders as they left for their jobs or came back from their shifts. Medical professionals and first responders were in high demand like never before; many sacrificed themselves and sacrificed time they could spend with family to take care of patients in the hospitals. This was a great act of selflessness; working firsthand with COVID victims not only put their lives at risk but also there was the possibility that someone could take the virus home. This was a poignant reminder of Jesus's ultimate sacrifice for us all. He willingly sacrificed himself for the salvation and redemption of humanity:

> "Greater love has no one than this: to lay down one's life for one's friends" (John 15:13 NIV).

It was in January 2020 that I would really see my calling as a physician when the United States took notice of COVID-19. News stories about the infections in China cropped up in newspapers, and television media also took up the story. All sorts of reports were coming out of China that several cities—comprising up to twenty million people—were being isolated.

I have to tell you, we did know from past experience that new strains of viruses could crop up in China. We started speculating that these viruses could affect humans and could be carried by and mutate in animals. When this coronavirus sprang up in Wuhan, people noted that there was a wet market dealing in aquatic and land animals only four miles away from the Wuhan Institute of Virology. It's possible that in a wet market, viruses can move from one animal to another and then to a human handler. Then the human handler spreads it to other people. That's just a theory. I wasn't ready to accept that theory then or accept it now. No one really knew exactly how and where this SARS-CoV-2 developed. I think it's more than a coincidence that the Institute is in Wuhan, and the first cases we know of came from that city. So, I believe the laboratory did have something to do with it, likely from poor safety practices.

Ironically, in January 2020, people in the United States certainly did not fear the worst. Many were yet to fully grasp the magnitude of the impending crisis, the extent of its impact, and the potential global ramifications on health. When the first outbreak happened, it seemed like a China problem. The geographical distance gave the perception that the virus could not in any way reach the United States. There was also limited information on the virus, its severity, and how it spread. Truth and facts were withheld. Few people knew it had the potential to cause a worldwide pandemic. Not to mention, media coverage was not as alarming in the beginning as it should have been. This, in a way, downplayed the threat of the virus; additionally, many people in the United States believed the virus would not have such a broad impact in the United States, as the government had better resources to handle it.

It reminded me of a situation a few years before. It was a year when the seasonal flu shots were not particularly effective (flu vaccines must be manufactured in the spring, and the vaccine manufacturers must guess exactly what the flu virus configuration will be eight months later). The "guess" of the flu vaccine was off that year, and we had a bad flu winter. The vaccine was only about 25 percent effective; consequently, the flu killed nearly eighty thousand people in the United States. That was about as bad as we thought we would be likely to face if COVID-19 spread here. In that bad flu winter, there had been no lockdowns, and no one outside the surgery operating rooms wore masks.

Still, the reports about the new coronavirus from Wuhan were troubling enough in January that I was asked to discuss it on the *Tamron Hall* show in New York City to comment on these stories. I had done some television commentary while working in Arkansas and was called in for expert opinion. I am straightforward, do my research, and express firsthand from my own patient care experiences exactly what I believe is happening and where we are headed. When other media outlets also began contacting me to discuss the virus, I was glad to educate the public and express the cautions, the health symptoms, the safety measures, and what we can do to keep our families safe based on my hands-on experience with my COVID patients.

Like most people at the time, my hope was that this new coronavirus would be a problem mainly concentrated in China, but we also knew that modern air travel could spread the virus in hours to locations around the world. I made several points. At the time, there was only one confirmed case of the new coronavirus disease in the United States, in a man who was quarantined and recovering adequately. I reported that in Asia, most people who had contracted the disease were suffering flu-like symptoms and mainly recovered in a manner like recovering from the flu. But I also added that people with such conditions as asthma, diabetes, or heart disease would be at risk for more serious ailments, including viral-instigated pneumonia.

I urged caution, and I pointed out several behaviors people could do that would lower the odds of becoming infected. These behaviors were good for any viral threat, be it from flu or the common cold or, if the coronavirus spread significantly to the United States, from the new coronavirus disease. These recommendations will sound familiar enough: wash your hands, keep your fingers away from your face, get enough rest and eat well, stay away from people who are sick, and stay away from people if you do get sick. I also urged people to follow a healthy lifestyle, that is, no smoking, go easy on the alcohol, exercise and stay in shape. Tamron smartly asked me, "What does exercise and good nutrition have to do with COVID?" I replied that it strengthens your immune system, and thus it is more effective at fighting off infection. At the early time of the pandemic, it was standard, so there was no need to mention masks or isolation or wiping down items and so forth. That was to change big time.

There were some other things that troubled me. I had suspicions about a Chinese medical professional who seemed compelled by his moral compass to speak more openly about the coronavirus threat but who suddenly either died or disappeared. Another grave concern was that we in the United States medical profession were acutely aware that both Severe Acute Respiratory Symptom (SARS) and influenza A subtype H5N1 (bird flu)) had begun in China and then spread to create epidemics in other countries. If it happened twice before, by God, it could happen again.

I advised, "Don't panic." This was good advice early on and is even now. It's never helpful to panic. To panic is to waste precious energy that could be applied to finding solutions. Looking back, it was best to advise greater urgency for vulnerable populations and to prepare for what was to come for the world, the United States, and in particular, that early spring, New York City. I did not know. No one else knew either.

PRAYER

Father Lord, we pray that you may give us a heart of compassion and love for our neighbors. May we always consider others through our actions. Help us to always treat our neighbors as we would like to be treated, and may we give ourselves service to others.

REFLECTION

The greatest display of humanity is giving up oneself for the service of others. The selflessness demonstrated by healthcare providers and first responders was a profound lesson on the values of love, compassion, and caring for others as taught by Christ. Jesus Christ showed us an example through his ultimate sacrifice; he willingly gave up his life for the salvation and redemption of human beings. This reflects the ultimate act of love and devotion.

God also calls us to love our neighbors as we love ourselves. Always treat others as you would like to be treated, for it is only through this that we can embody Christ's teachings.

ECHOES OF SUFFERING: THE LINGERING EFFECTS OF COVID'S WRATH

March 2020 was the most extraordinary medical month modern New York City had ever suffered. The city had its first confirmed COVID-19 case on March 1, though we had suspected a few cases in February and even in January. Although we were hoping the virus could be contained in China, we saw in February that it had spread to other places, most notably Italy. I knew that if the virus was spreading in Italy, it would be challenging to keep it out of the United States. And if it were to come to the United States from Italy and Europe, it would most likely enter through the busiest East Coast airports, that is, through the three regional New York airports: JFK, LaGuardia, and Newark.

We were right. It was coming at us. Unfortunately, we had little to use in our own defense. Initially, we did not have test kits with which to test for COVID-19 infections. People came to our health center with coughs, sneezes, and fever, but without proper testing kits, we could not be sure if they had colds or COVID-19. We were able to test for flu. I recall my first patient who came in with a high fever; I was hoping he would test positive for influenza versus COVID and he did. We were all relieved. All we could do was provide supportive care—give cough medicine for coughs and Tylenol or Motrin for fever and pain. We advised patients to stay hydrated and gave inhalers to people with trouble breathing, but that was about it. It wasn't until much later, and as the disease began ravaging people, families, and communities, that more supplies and equipment came that could help us diagnose the condition, ease symptoms, and work against transmission from infected to uninfected people.

However, we were still early in the year and had little medicine with which to work beyond palliative care. We were hit with a sucker punch as the city's first confirmed case came on March 1. A very bad sign came in the second week of the month: the disease was spreading rapidly here, here in New York City. Oh, my good God. New York City is very densely populated. Moreover, New Yorkers are out-and-about creatures; they come, go, and interact—in business meetings, in movies, live theaters, sports stadiums, schools, and museums. They packed themselves densely in office building lobbies, elevators, subways, and buses. Our city was a very fertile territory—a hot bed, no pun intended—for this kind of viral transmission. Matching our worst fears, within days, our magnificent New York City was now the epicenter of the deadly coronavirus disease in the United States.

On March 16, the city closed its public schools, and the state closed its colleges and universities. On March 20, Governor Cuomo's office sent a stay-at-home order and closed all nonessential businesses. Astonishingly, New York City streets began to look deserted, as if they were scenes from a science-fiction disaster movie. The fear was spreading fast; people were starting to realize the virus's global health impact. Some people made a lot of poor decisions based on their fears; but remember the Lord tells us in Isaiah 41:10 NIV, "So do not fear, for I am with you; do not be dismayed, for I am your God. I will strengthen you and help you; I will uphold you with my righteous right hand."

At this time, medical staff were told not to dress as we usually do in our "civilian clothes." We were asked to wear N95 masks, gloves, and full gowns. We were dressing for battle with an invisible enemy. We started wearing face shields. I wore them almost 24/7. I do think they helped protect me from contracting the disease. I needed to help save lives; I couldn't afford to get sick; I certainly couldn't call in sick. It was hard to breathe in those astronaut uniforms, but it was necessary. I was in and around COVID all day long.

Did the school and business mandates and shutdowns prevent viral human-to-human transmissions? The blow to New York was severe. By the end of March, we had had more than thirty thousand cases, making the city the worst-hit anywhere in the country. Six days into April, New York City had more COVID-19 cases than the officially reported cases in China, the UK, and Iran *combined.* Our city had already recorded two thousand deaths. Bodies of those who had died were being picked up by US Army soldiers and members of the New York Army National Guard. Refrigeration trucks had been rushed to New York hospital parking lots to hold bodies as morgues. Because hospital beds and rooms became filled, field hospitals—essentially tents—were set up in several places, including Central Park. President Trump provided everything for us that our Governor Cuomo asked for. This helped me tremendously to do my job and care for my patients.

Increasing numbers of people streamed into our healthcare center. To state the obvious, we were not prepared for this. Our lobbies grew packed with people sick coughing and sneezing. Naturally, that is a lousy situation for viral spread. However, the public still had not been adequately informed about social transmission, nor could we have done much about keeping people ten feet apart in our packed lobbies. Nor could we have done anything about our ventilation system, which circulated the air and removed particulates but was not designed to trap viruses as small as SARS-CoV-2.

During this March-April period, we were hit with multiple problems at once. For one, the hospitals filled up. That meant that people with other ailments—chest pain that could signal an impending heart attack or abdominal pain that could be a symptom of appendicitis—could not receive the quick analysis and treatment they otherwise would have. In addition, the uncertainty and the economic downturn gave rise to crime, drug addiction, anorexia, mental illness, and suicide. All these required the attention of psychiatrists, healthcare staff, and public safety personnel, and all of these people were working overtime dealing with the escalating COVID-19 pandemic. This indeed gave cause to burnout fatigue or emotional distress among healthcare workers; it was always right around the corner because we couldn't see any relief ahead.

During such life difficulties, we put our faith and trust in God. We had reached a point where the frustration was palpable, we were being overwhelmed in hospitals, and the pandemic was only spreading wider, yet there was no foreseeable relief. When life feels impossible, we should turn to the God of possibilities. Psalm 34:17–18 NIV says, "The righteous cry out, and the Lord hears them; he delivers them from all their troubles."

The ravages of the virus weighed down many families—not only physically but emotionally, economically, and spiritually too. Some had lost hope and had grown weary of ever gaining a sense of normalcy again. Some people could not handle the weight of the impact and ended up committing suicide. We should not let the world's weight pull us down when the Lord promises to walk with us and always give us rest whenever we seek Him. In Matthew 11:28–30 NIV He says,

"Come to me, all you who are weary and burdened, and I will give you rest. Take my yoke upon you and learn from me, for I am gentle and humble in heart, and you will find rest for your souls."

Everyone everywhere—and especially in healthcare facilities such as the one where I worked—had to work long, long hours. Our days became exhausting. By the end of March, about 90 percent of my patients were COVID-19-related patients or suspected to have been infected with the coronavirus. In one shift, I saw ninety-four patients at West 39th Street. My feet were numb at the end of the shift, and my legs ached horribly. I was exhausted, and on top of this, some of my friends and family members were dying. It was truly horrible, and what I was experiencing was mirrored in all the medical staff at our facility. During this time, I could comfort myself with the word of God as He says in 2 Corinthians 4:16–18 ESV, "So, we do not lose heart. Though our outer self is wasting away, our inner self is being renewed day by day. For this light momentary affliction is preparing for us an eternal weight of glory beyond all comparison, as we look not to the things that are seen but to the things that are unseen. For the things that are seen are transient, but the things that are unseen are eternal."

I believed these words strongly in my heart; there had to be something better coming. I refused to believe this was our forever reality because if I did, I would have lost my mind. By shifting my perspective and focusing on the glory of God and the good He had in store for us, I could show up each day and give my best to my patients.

What physical and mental rest we could get was a fitful sleep, which was always too short and followed directly by going right back into the medical exam rooms, like going back to the battlefront, where we faced anxious patients. They were scared; people couldn't breathe, people were dying. There was a time paramedics did not perform CPR due to the risk of COVID exposure if the patient at home had no pulse.

Rumors flew. I recall one woman screaming at me not to send her husband to Elmhurst Hospital—the closest available hospital to the healthcare facility where I worked—because at Elmhurst "everybody died." Her husband desperately needed oxygen, which Elmhurst had, and we ran out. Our oxygen tanks were empty, but she was convinced Elmhurst was merely a place where patients went to die.

Keep in mind, in the beginning, we medical staff on the front lines of care had very little with which to fight this awful pandemic. As noted, initially we had few tests for SARS-CoV-2, and for coronavirus infections, there really were no significant treatments. We did have a test for the flu, so if someone came in with flu-like symptoms, we gave them that test. If the test showed the patient had the flu, I was relieved; there's not much you can do for the flu except antivirals and supportive care like hot tea with honey, fever/pain meds, and wait, but at least the patient did not have COVID-19. I would give out free samples of ibuprofen and natural vitamins like BC BOOST (a proprietary combination of vitamins I developed myself), which contains vitamin D3 and zinc, shown to help with infections and boost your immune system along with vitamins C and B12. BC BOOST indeed supported their health. Later on, studies came out showing the immense value of vitamins D and C for COVID and other viral illnesses too. During March and April, one way we could "test" for COVID-19 when we ran out of nasal swabs was a chest X-ray. That's because we learned that patients with COVID-19 had a rather distinctive pattern showing up in their X-rays. Their X-rays resembled snow, as if someone had thrown a snowball that had splattered across their lungs—that is what the COVID-19 pneumonia looked like. I recognized it instantly on X-rays. In the beginning, that was our "test." It wasn't conclusive, but it was practically all we had, and it helped a lot until we got more nasal swabs available.

We began to feel desperate as more and more patients came in with COVID-19 symptoms, and as more New Yorkers were dying, and the morgues overflowed with bodies. I thought my time working natural disasters was horrific until the pandemic hit, and I pledged to stay alive and help as many others as I could. I cried sometimes. I didn't let anyone see me cry…but I did. The support of my awesome family, my dear friends, and my amazing colleagues at Fox always lifted me, reaching out with love and checking up on me. One of my best friends, Mark, knowing I grew up on an orange grove in Florida, would drop off Florida navel oranges while I was working. They were delicious. My TV colleagues were so supportive: a text from Ainsley to stay safe or a note of encouragement from David always put a smile on my face. This kindness motivated me and my staff and was a reminder that God has blessed me to become a doctor, and I will always be grateful and cherish the privilege to care for others.

In the beginning, for a brief time, we prescribed hydroxychloroquine off label. This was a medicine taken in pill form that is used to help prevent and treat malaria, certain types of lupus, and rheumatoid arthritis. Hydroxychloroquine is thought useful in these cases because it kills malaria protozoa that cause malaria and counters lupus and rheumatoid arthritis because it suppresses some activities of the immune system. At the end of March, the FDA approved the use of hydroxychloroquine for patients hospitalized with COVID-19. But three months later, the FDA recommended against using it because patients who were prescribed hydroxychloroquine did not do better than those who did not take it, but it was worth trying if it could potentially save lives[1]. Some of my patients said it helped, some did not. President Trump was given this medication by his doctor after he was exposed to COVID by his security team. This was a moment in history where we should have robustly tested the use of existing medications to treat or minimize COVID. We had nothing to lose other than life—risk versus benefit.

---

1 U.S. Food and Drug Administration. "FDA Cautions Against Use of Hydroxychloroquine or Chloroquine for COVID-19 Outside of the Hospital Setting or a Clinical Trial Due to Risk of Heart Rhythm Problems." FDA, April 24, 2020. https://www.fda.gov/drugs/drug-safety-and-availability/fda-cautions-against-use-hydroxychloroquine-or-chloroquine-covid-19-outside-hospital-setting-or.

At least by this point in time, we got all the equipment we needed at our healthcare facility: gowns, masks, and face shields to stop the direct transmission of the virus from one patient through the air to a healthcare worker nearby. We also had an excess of ventilators. But what we did not have was enough staff to handle the load of patients. There was such a shortage that even orthopedic surgeons were asked to help, despite it not being their specialty. Most people who came in had COVID-19 symptoms but not so severe that they needed to go to a hospital. Most could be sent home with inhalers, fever meds, and instructions on how to weather through the week to recover. We lacked medical professionals to see them, listen to them, diagnose them, and tell them how best to endure the infection at home and not infect others. There just weren't enough healthcare providers for that.

As time went on, we learned more about the coronavirus. Two strains of coronavirus—alpha and beta—cause the common cold. But the novel coronavirus, COVID-19, has receptor projections that not only attach to cells in our noses like the alpha and beta ones do but also to tissues in our lungs. COVID-19 viruses target the lungs, and then people have trouble breathing; their blood oxygen goes down, and in severe cases, they must be put on ventilators, which provide oxygen into the lungs. If the lung infection is serious enough, the patient cannot absorb enough oxygen, resulting in organ failure and death. When we see people coming in with symptoms, we hope their oxygen levels are ninety-eight or ninety-nine, which is the level for healthy persons. But we were seeing people with levels below eighty, and we'd put them on oxygen to try to get those levels back above ninety.

Sometimes it was a real struggle. I was seeing patients with seriously low oxygen levels—in the seventies and eighties. About 20 percent of the patients we were seeing had to be admitted to the hospitals and be intubated, that is, put on a ventilator to help them breathe. During the spring of 2020, this was serious; indeed, about 80 percent of those intubated died. Word got out, and people were naturally scared to go to hospitals for fear of being put on a ventilator. They died at home. Even medical staff came to fear ventilators. I had a colleague who came down with COVID-19 and told his doctors, "Don't intubate me. Just put me on the high-flow oxygen mask." He came very close to dying but survived. Nevertheless, the common practice at the time was to intubate seriously ill patients. Now we don't jump to ventilators as we used to because we didn't know much about this virus and its origin. It seemed like those on ventilators died. We would rather put them on high-flow oxygen to keep them alive. Hospitals use ventilators only as a very last resort.

PRAYER

Almighty God, we pray that you may give us the strength to push through our difficult and challenging times. We are weak and sinful; we cannot overcome life's troubles without your help. Send your Holy Spirit, the helper, to help us in our times of need. Restore our faith in your word, that we may never lose hope in life. Amen.

REFLECTION

In this reflection, we focus on human beings' response to challenges and difficulties in their lives. It is important to note that having a strong faith does not exempt you from experiencing difficulties in life. And even though faith gives people a strong foundation to handle most things, the realities of life can still test you in a way you are not prepared for. The Bible is full of stories from firm believers who faced hard times, but through their trust in God, they came out victorious. The story of Job's suffering is one of the many stories that underscore the reality that believers, too, can face hardships. Having faith does not promise you a life free from suffering, but if you suffer in Christ, you will receive the glory of God. To navigate the storms of life, ground yourself in the teachings of Christ and cultivate a deeper understanding of His promises.

UNMASKING COVID-19 FACTS AND MYTHS

Spring of 2020 was also a busy time because I was reporting daily or weekly for Fox News. I was all about science, the facts, and the data and talking about my real-life, hands-on patient experiences and sharing them with the nation and the world. I emphasized the basics: washing hands, rest, nutrition, staying away from people if you are coughing or sneezing. I encouraged people to follow local guidelines provided by the government and health officials in their area. To those still traveling, I advised them to check travel advisories and follow CDC safety measures, which at that time included wearing masks, areas of good ventilation, and maintaining safe distance from those who were sick. There was also a lot of misinformation going around during this period. I encouraged people to rely on trustworthy sources of information such as your doctor or the daily Health Department news briefs to stay updated on the latest developments.

They say sometimes prevention is better than a cure; for a virus that we had yet to figure out, these preventive measures were the best steps we could take at that time. Those who took heed and implemented these measures survived the worst of it. Those who did not may have struggled. Even the Bible warns us about the consequences of not staying away from danger. Proverbs 22:3 NIV says, "The prudent see danger and take refuge, but the simple keep going and pay the penalty."

We soon began hearing a lot of talk about "flattening the curve." This was in reference to the projected rise and fall of infections, which made a rising and falling line shaped somewhat like a bell curve. Television news shows generally showed two projections: first, a steep and narrow bell curve and second, a lower, flatter, broader bell curve. At the time, what we were working toward—and what we were telling people to work toward—was the flatter curve, indicating a reduction in infection. Why? Because we didn't want the healthcare system to collapse in chaos. We couldn't take care of one thousand patients at once, but we could take care of one hundred at once.

According to the science, and the reason for wanting a broader, flatter bell curve, is that if the infection experience was a steep rise—even if followed by a steep fall—the number of infected and sick people would overwhelm hospital space. With full hospitals—that is, with overflowing lobbies and bed space at capacity—a number of bad things would happen. For one, even when a hospital is fully staffed, if the hospital is full, the staff is stressed and stretched to the limit, physically and emotionally. That means individual patients cannot receive the targeted care—medical and emotional—that they really need. Second, the staff themselves will get sick. That means the sick ones have to stay home—assuming their symptoms are mild enough to keep themselves out of hospital beds—and that makes it even harder for the remaining working staff to care for patients. Given the conditions in New York City at the time, a very steep rise in infections would most certainly lead to increased deaths—and we were having far too many deaths as it was, including dying nurses and even doctors and first responders.

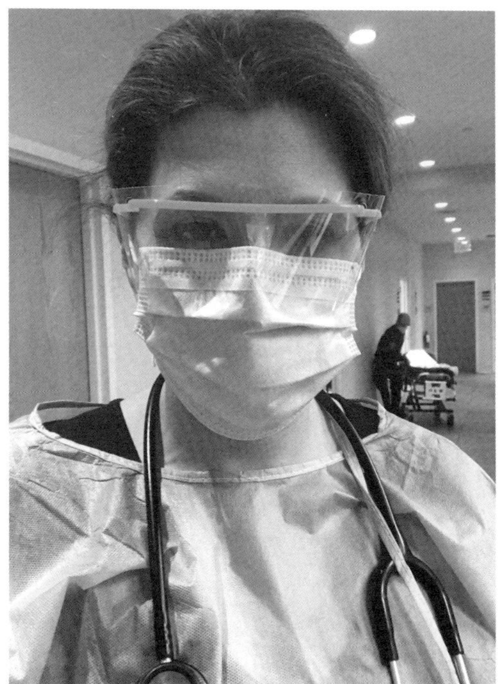

Taking care of Covid Patients in full PPE gear.

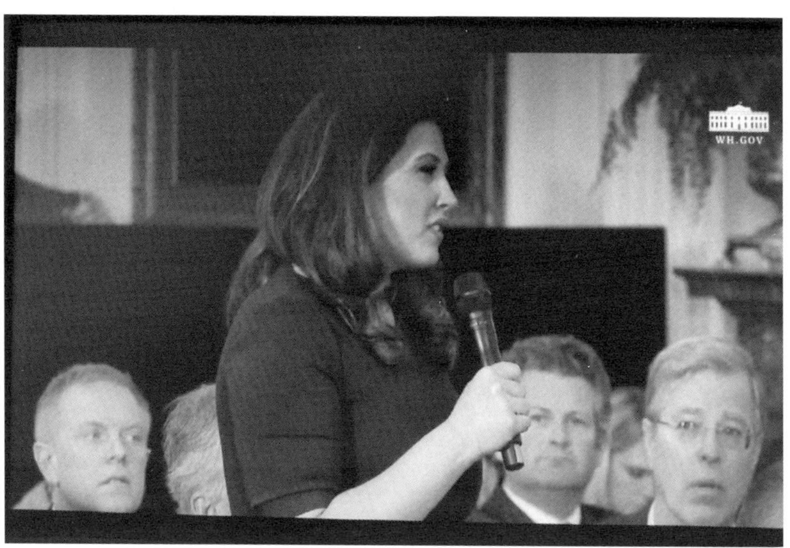

Speaking at the White House Opioid Summit in Washington, DC.

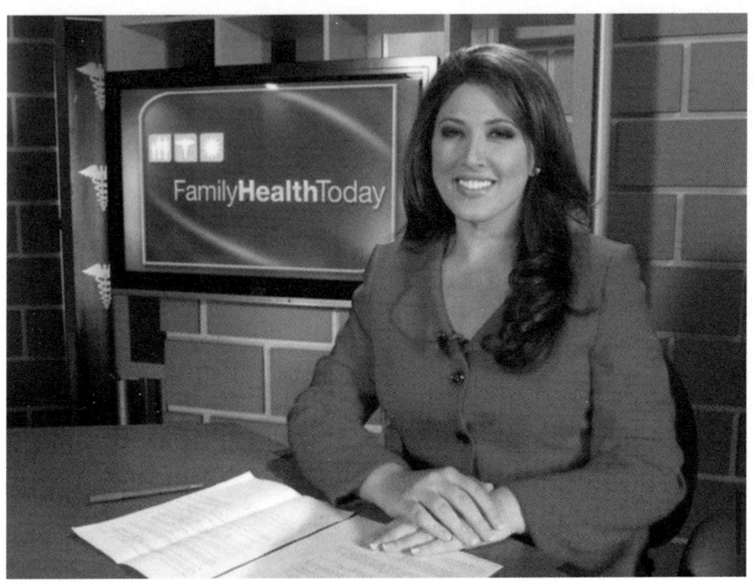

Hosting my first solo TV Health Program while in medical residency, *Family Health Today.*

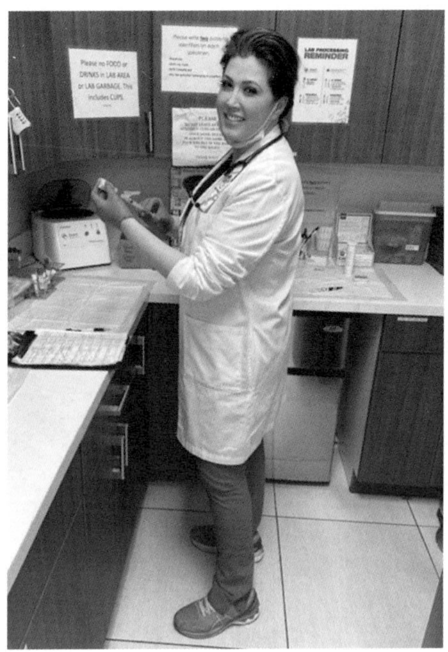

Drawing up penicillin for a patient.

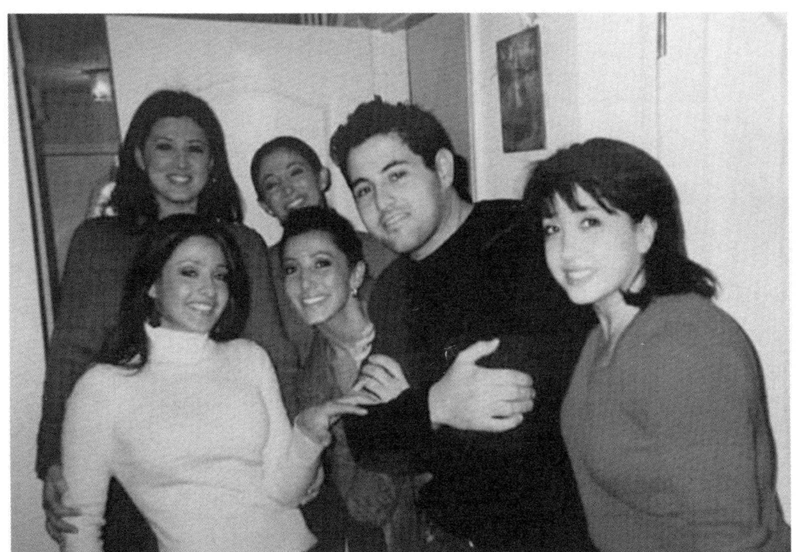

My Mom and Siblings.

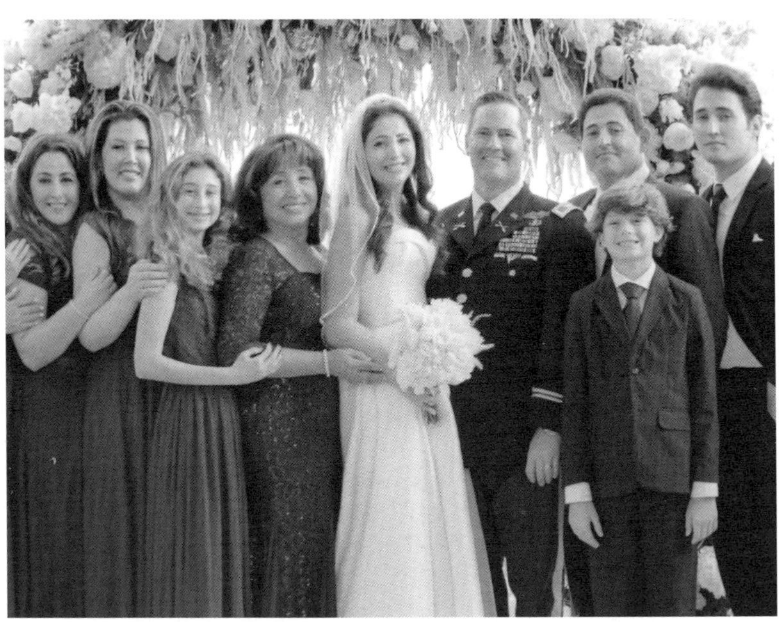

A Family Wedding is a family reunion: my sister, Captain Julia Nesheiwat.

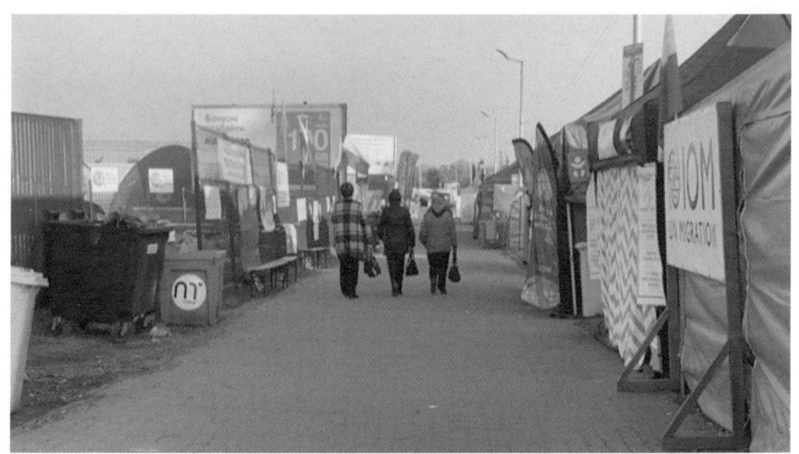

Refugees fleeing Ukraine.

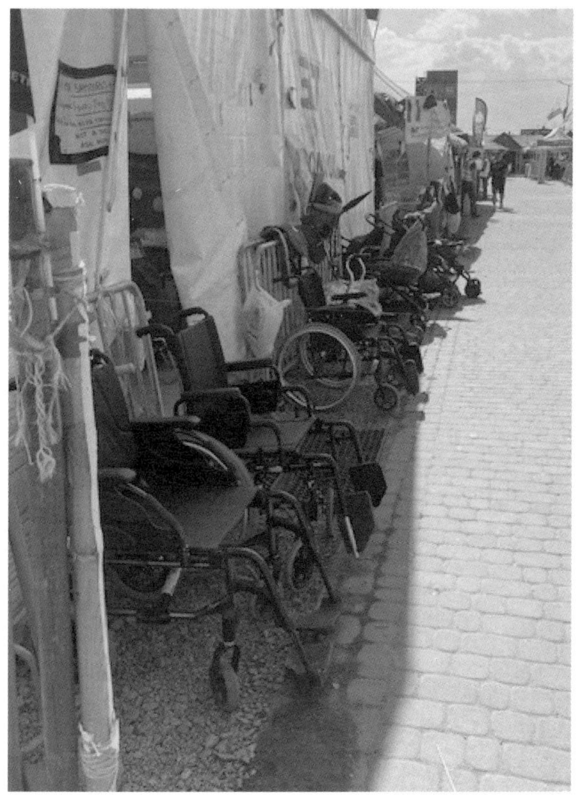

Wheelchairs for those who could not walk due to bombings from Russian Attacks.

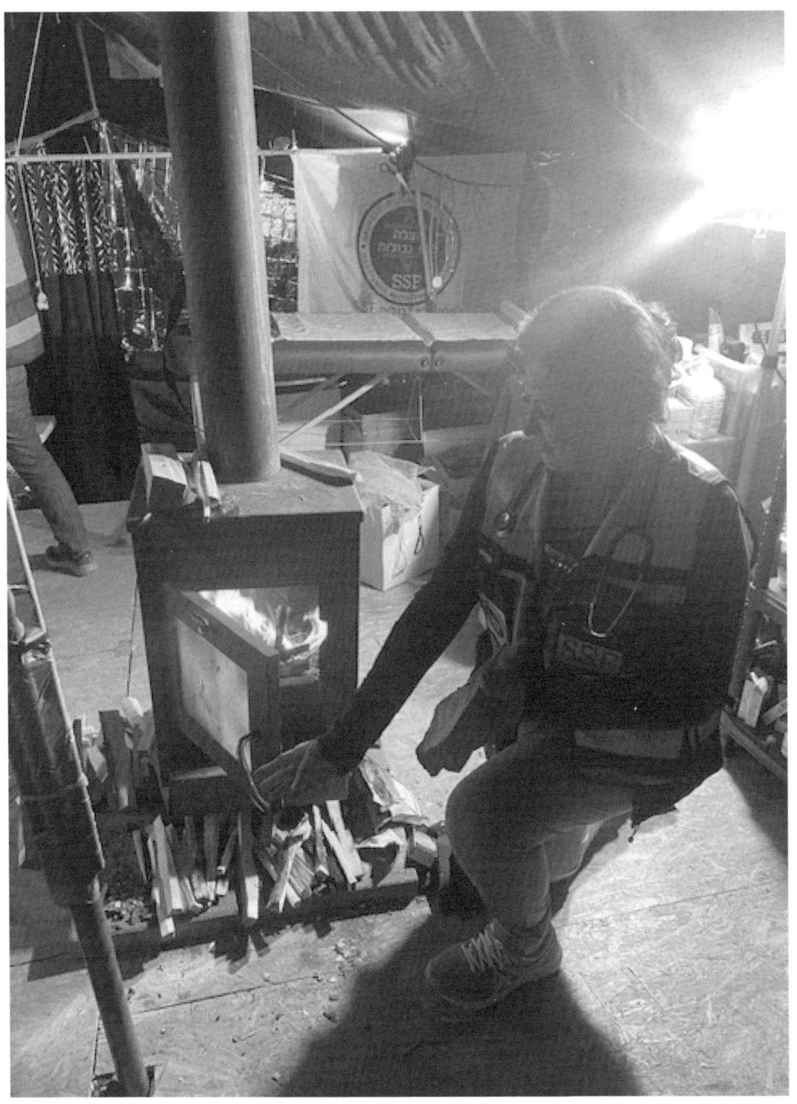

Trying to keep warm while caring for Ukrainians at the Polish border, we chopped wood to keep the fire going throughout the night.

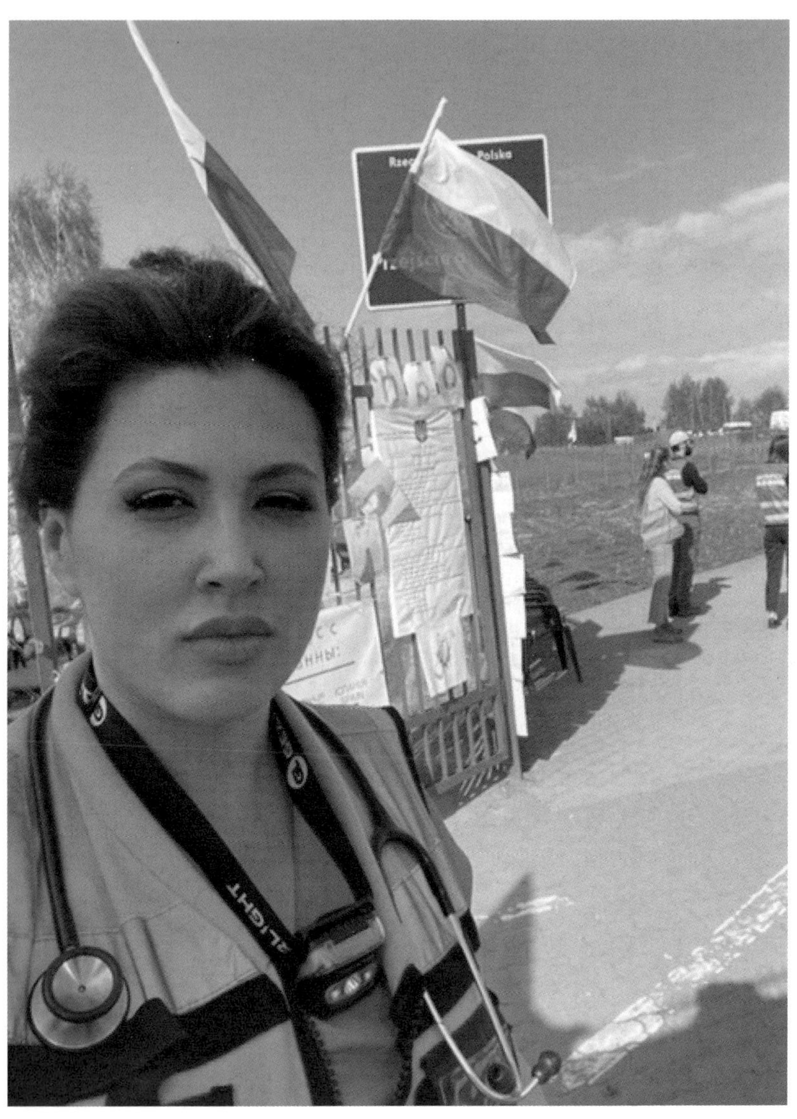

Working at the Ukrainian border caring for injured and ill Ukrainians.

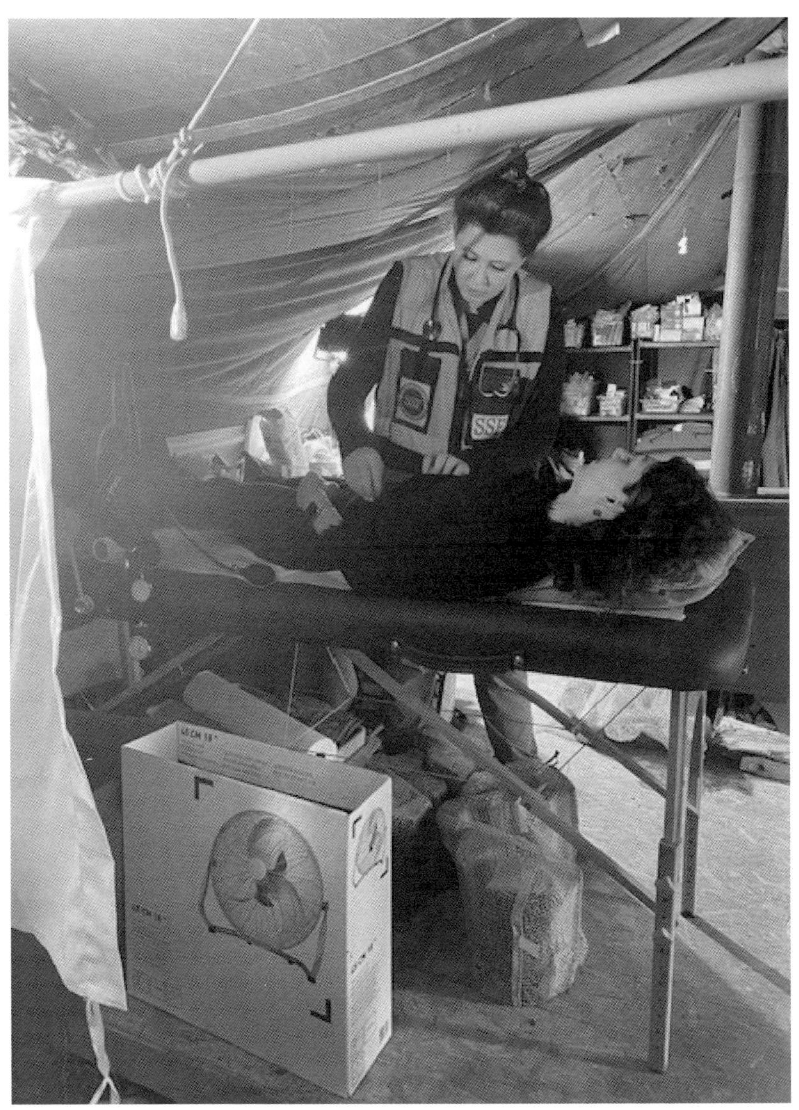

Examining an assaulted female in a tent at the Ukraine border of Medyka.

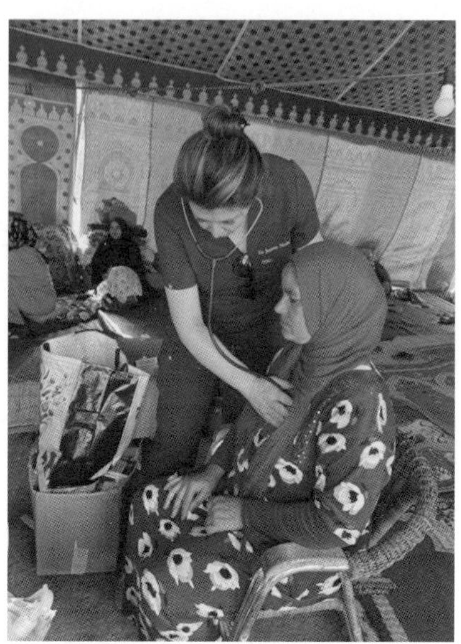

Caring for patients after the Moroccan earthquake.

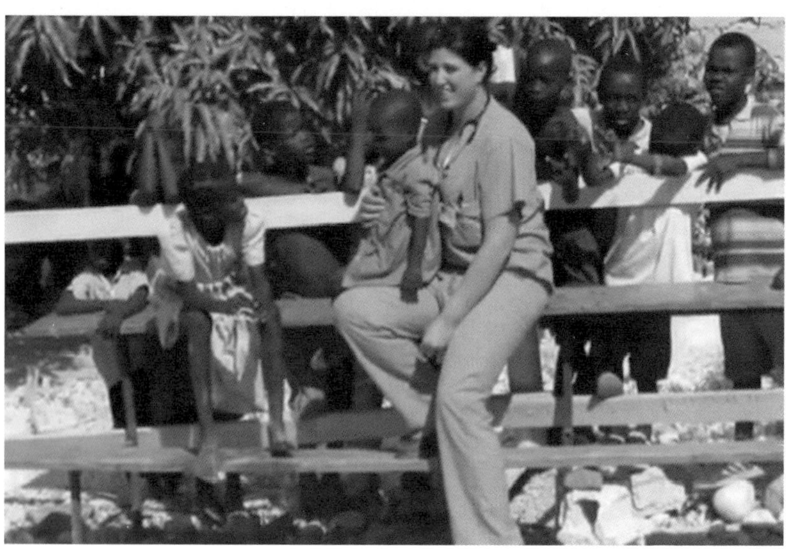

Providing medical care for children after the earthquake at the Ebenezer Orphanage in Haiti.

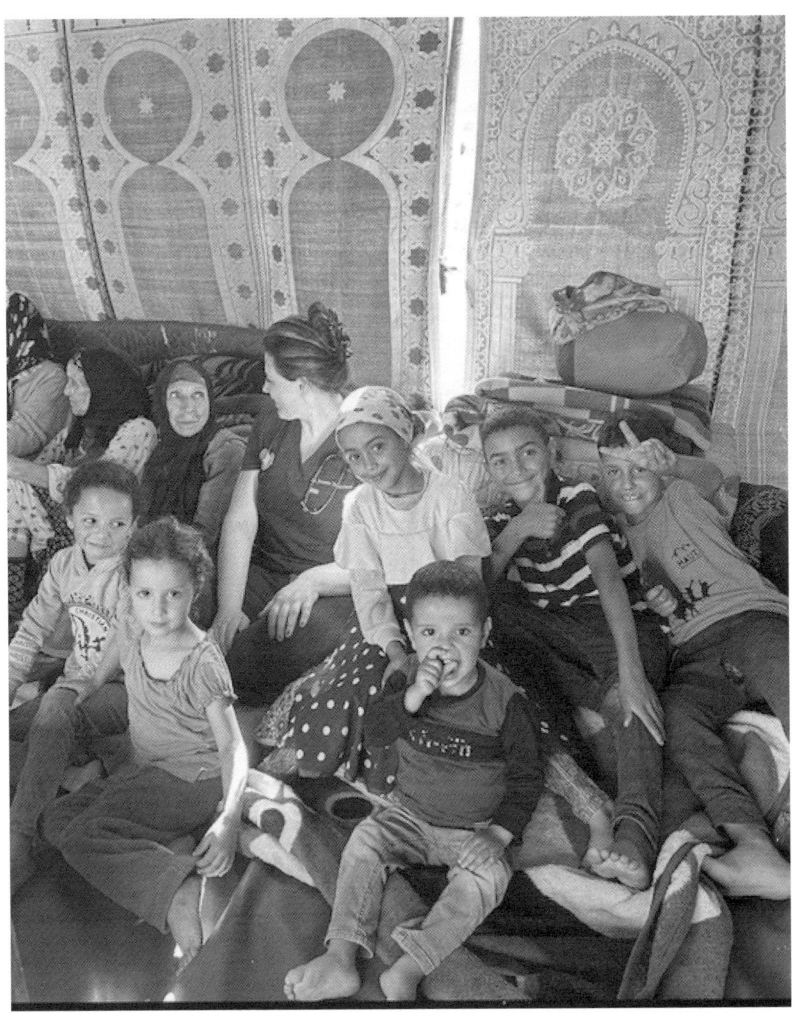

Orphaned Moroccan children after the earthquake struck in Africa.

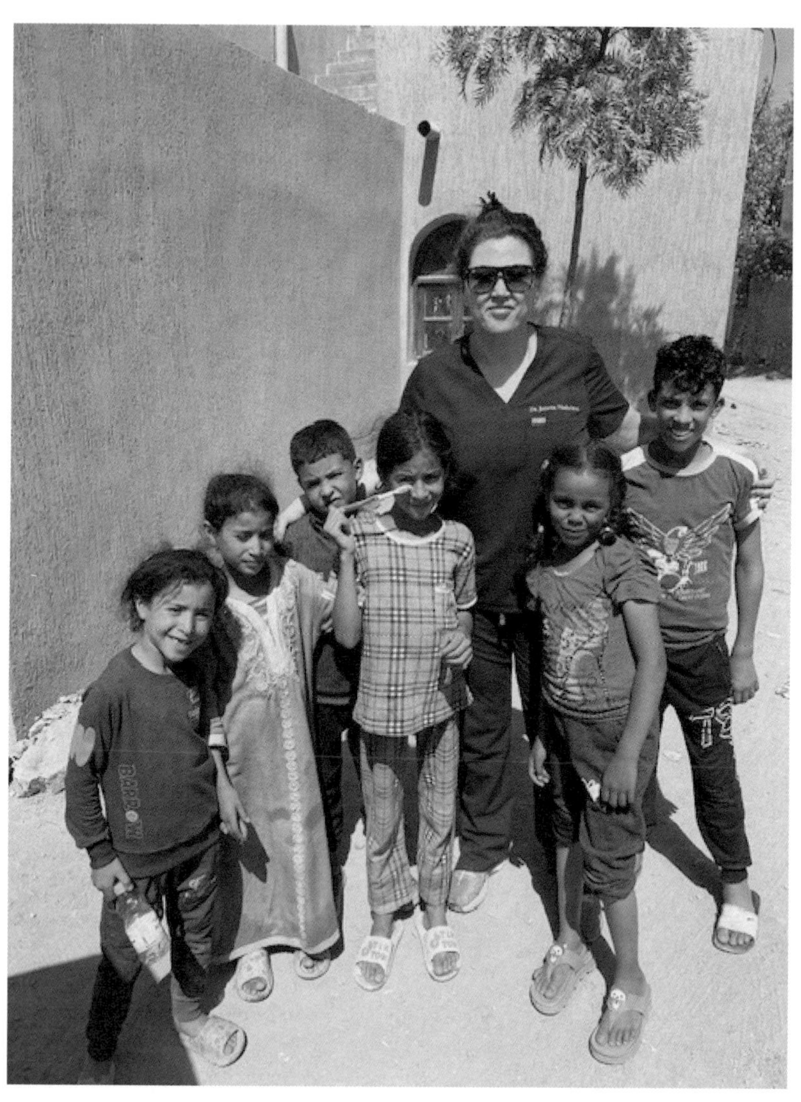

Providing medical care and food for Moroccan children in the Atlas mountains post-earthquake.

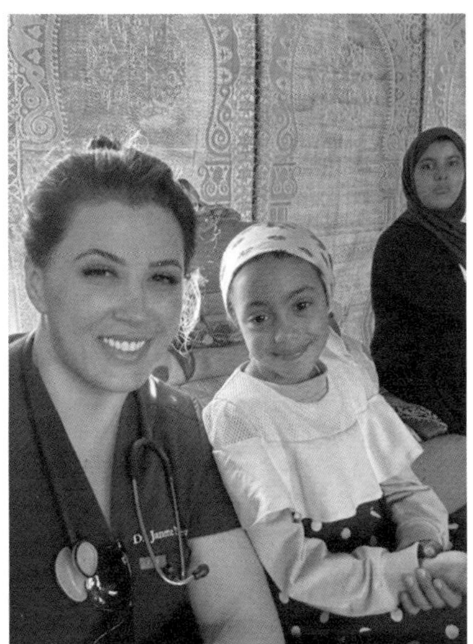

Trying to cheer up a little girl who lost her mom after the Moroccan earthquake near Marrakech.

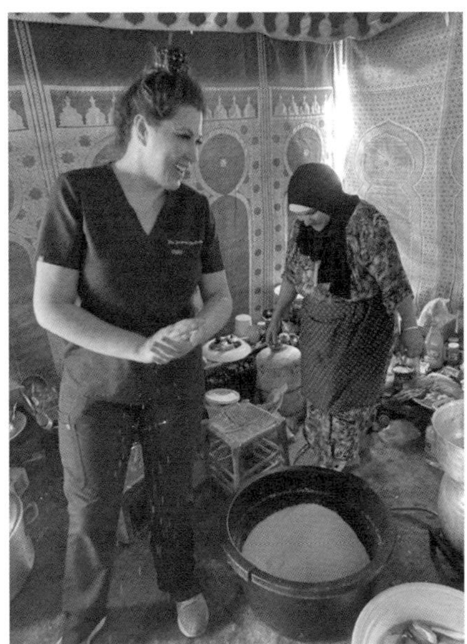

In the village of the Atlas Mountains of Morocco, where I was asked to pray for the meal.

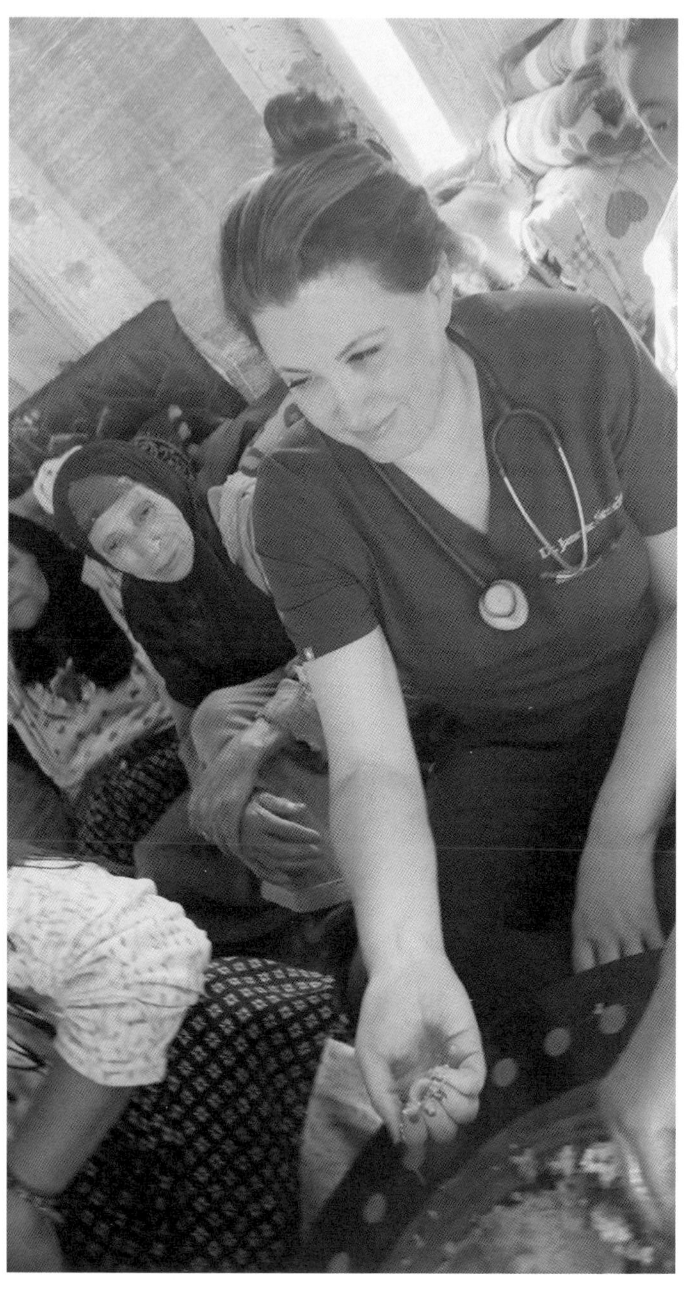

Having couscous with the survivors of the earthquake in Africa, tradition to eat with one's hand.

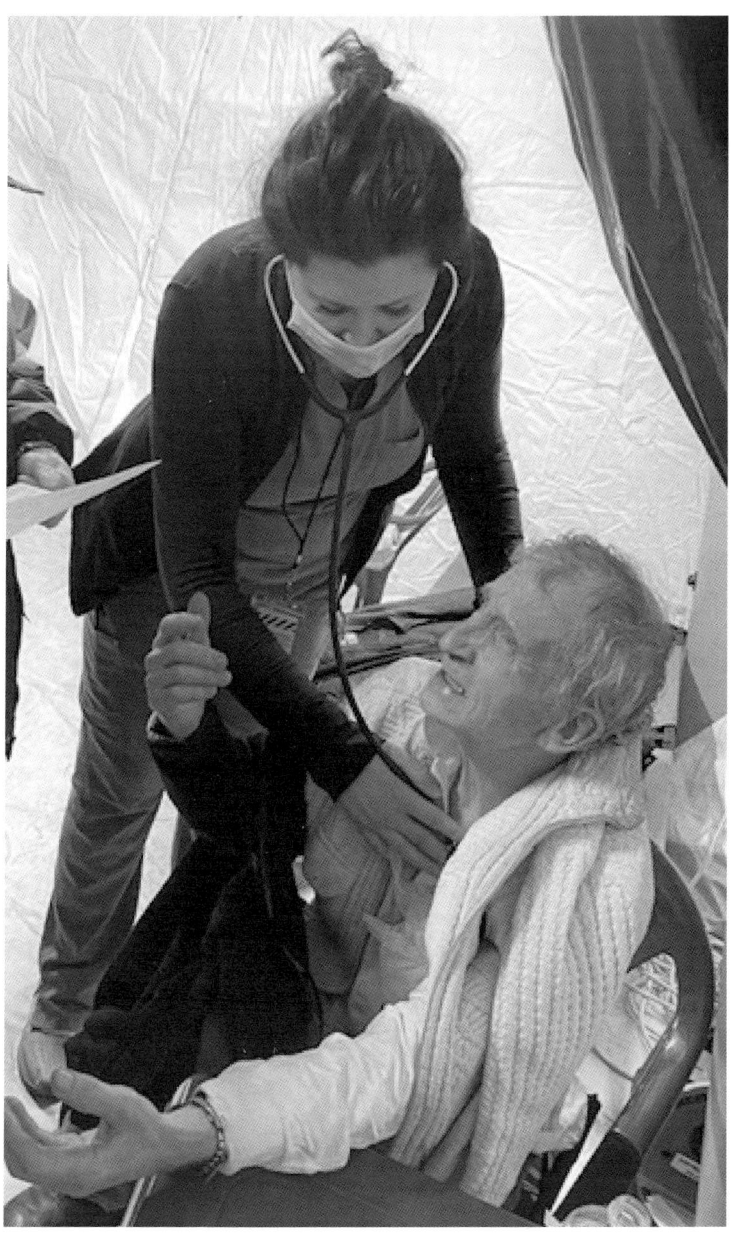

In Lviv, Ukraine examining a Ukrainian refugee who fled Kherson suffering from a heart attack after the Russian invasion.

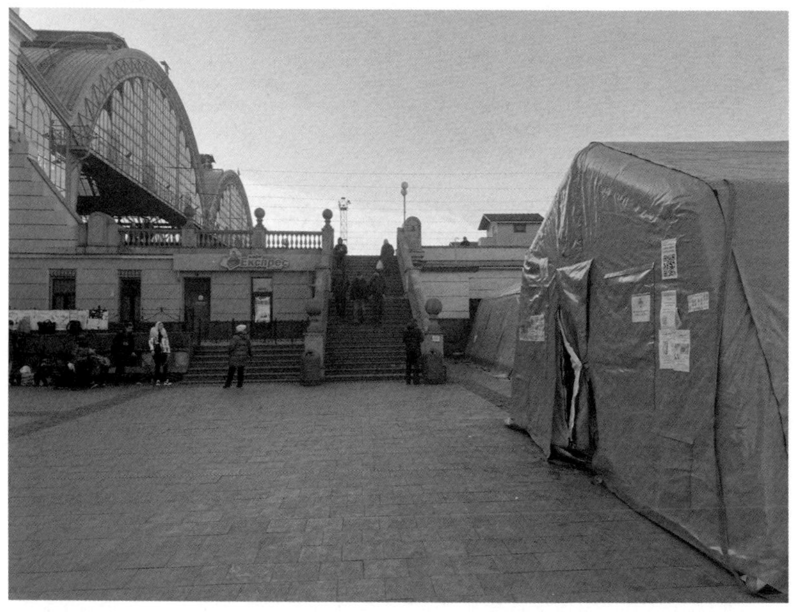

The base of the Lviv Railway in Ukraine where we set up a makeshift tent to care for injured and ill Ukrainians.

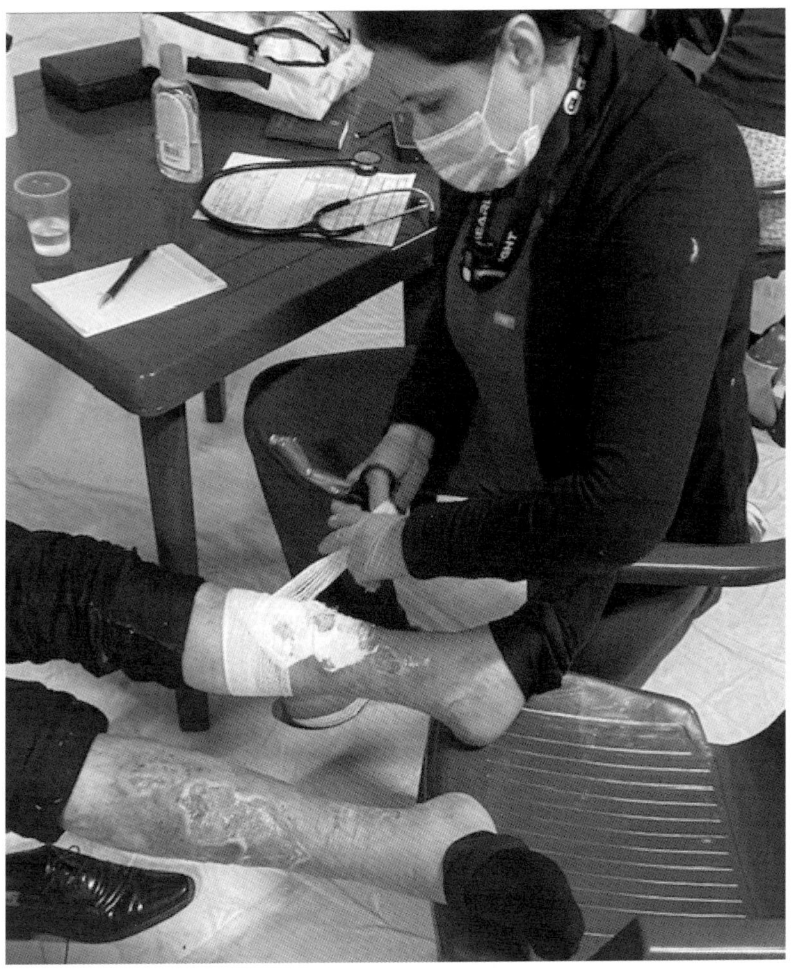

Providing wound care for a burn patient in Ukraine who injured his legs in an explosion by a Russian attack.

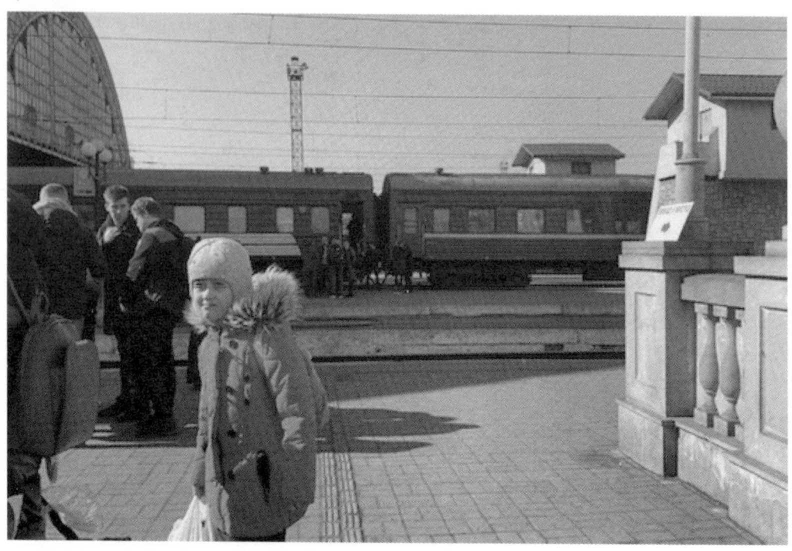

The tender glance of a young child fleeing Ukraine to safety.

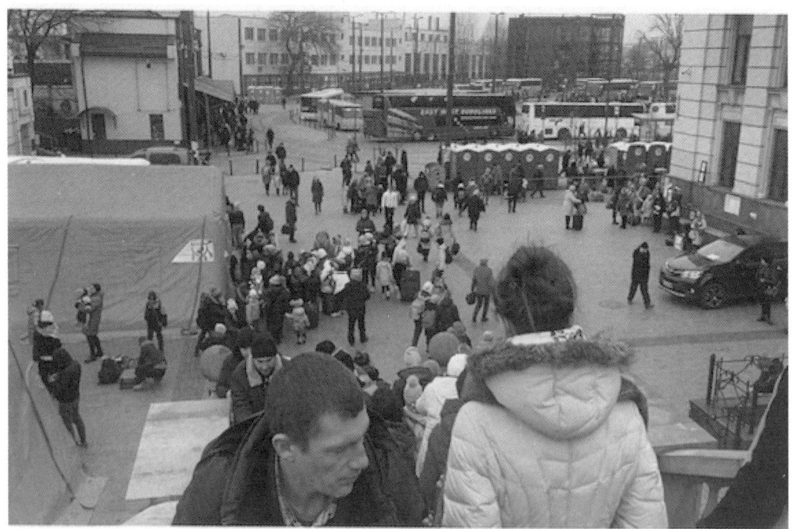

The Lviv Railway in Ukraine where many were fleeing Ukraine after the Russian attack and seeking medical care.

So, the remedy was to "flatten the curve," meaning to slow the number of infections. Given that a certain number of infections were going to take place anyway, a lower peak and a broader bell curve would mean that the duration of the infection period would be longer, but the strain on the hospital system at any given time would be lower and more spread out. This is what we were looking for at the time. And this is what Dr. Fauci and other national experts were advocating.

I reported on TV news honestly, clearly, and completely. I always aimed for truth and compassion, and I made doubly sure that my coronavirus reports met that standard. People were getting very anxious, and at a time like that, they could pick up misinformation that could be harmful to them, and that could lead to panic. There were rumors about supposed miracle cures or treatments for COVID-19, leading some individuals to pursue unproven and potentially harmful remedies instead of seeking proper medical care. Some theories suggested that the virus was intentionally created and spread for political reasons. Naturally, this led some people to mistrust the public health system; therefore, they were skeptical. Further confusion about how the virus originated and spread may have led to more people contracting the virus. The truth at the beginning could have saved lives. Many people ended up dying due to a lack of proper knowledge or getting the correct information, which is why I took it upon myself to ensure I educated as many people as I could on the virus based on what I was seeing on the front lines, in the trenches with my own COVID patients. The Bible says in Hosea 4:6 NKJV, "My people are destroyed for lack of knowledge; because you have rejected knowledge, I reject you from being a priest to me. And since you have forgotten the law of your God, I also will forget your children."

Still, everyone felt anxious, some even frantic. The people we worked with, our healthcare colleagues, were getting sick. It wasn't difficult to figure out why; we were working with COVID-19 patients every day. Many of us had to stay at work or in the area, not seeing our family for days. We worried we would bring the virus home to our families. This was at a period when people were not going out much or going out only when they really had to. And they were wiping down anything they brought home from a store, even bags or cans or bottles.

Personally, I didn't want to infect my family, so I painstakingly stayed away from them at the beginning of the pandemic. My mom lives in Tennessee, and though we talk nearly every day, I stopped my monthly visits because I knew, as an older person, she was more vulnerable to serious complications stemming from the disease. When I did finally visit her, about a year into the pandemic, I was so emotionally moved to see her sitting in her chair when she looked up at me in such surprise, I fell to my knees at her feet, holding her so tightly. I missed her touch, and with tears streaming down my face, I reflected on the long, hard quarantine year being on the front line, facing death each day. I was really so happy and lucky she was alive. She never caught COVID, although everyone else in the house did. I tested myself before seeing her and wore my mask around her to keep her safe. She told me how she watched Fox News almost 24/7 to see and hear me speak.

Early in the pandemic, I would film right out of the TV station studio, but as the pandemic progressed and fear grew stronger, the new safety directive to all Fox News contributors was not to come to the studio at all but rather Skype or film from home or the hospital. I was mostly at work and hardly ever home, so I would sometimes film directly from the healthcare facility where

I worked. I set up a tripod from the clinic corridor or one of the patient exam rooms.

As the environment heated up, *Fox and Friends* asked me to report just about every day, wanting to know about my daily patient care, what I was experiencing, what I saw, about the environment, treatment, supplies, death rate, and so on. I may have been one of the few hands-on people regularly reporting on television who was actually treating the deluge of COVID-19 patients in NYC. I told it like I saw it. I did not hold back. It was raw and honest reporting. I wasn't just an agency head, or nonprofit leader, or a virologist. I was working on the front line, on site, reporting firsthand, and being at risk of being exposed to hundreds of COVID-infected patients of all ages and genders, acute, chronic, and dying.

Fox News wanted authentic reports directly out of the exam rooms from doctors who were actually testing and diagnosing patients, taking temperatures, taking blood pressure, and checking oxygen levels. They wanted to know the truth and the facts: what were the most common symptoms, what age groups seemed to have the worst or the mildest cases, what comorbidities such as obesity, diabetes, asthma, or heart trouble made the most severe cases, whether smokers suffered more than nonsmokers, whether overweight patients had more severe cases than slimmer ones, whether people with certain kinds of jobs or certain kinds of habits had worse cases, and so on. I gave answers as truthfully and completely as time and my own observations and care of patients allowed. I was exhausted but happy because the enormous feedback indicated people were listening, and my hope was to help save lives through educating.

PRAYER

Dear Lord, we pray that you may use us as vessels of truth; where there is misinformation, may we provide facts. We pray for the virtue of honesty. May our words always be truthful and trustworthy. Help us to lead people on the correct path when we see them being led astray. May we always seek your knowledge and be guided in it forever. Amen.

REFLECTION

Where do you get your information from? Just like a lot of misinformation spread during COVID, there is a lot of misinformation about what it means to believe in God. Without the proper knowledge and information, it is easy to be swayed by this misinformation and be led astray. As a Christian, it is essential to know God and experience Him for yourself; you can do this by reading the word of God and following His teachings. When you know the word of God, it is not easy to fall victim to false interpretations of the Bible. Jesus is the way, the truth, and the life—follow Him, and you will not be led astray.

PANDEMIC POLITICS: NAVIGATING THE POLITICAL MINEFIELD OF COVID-19

Unfortunately, medicine became politicized. This developed especially about a year into the pandemic when masking policies became controversial, and the vaccines became available thanks to Operation Warp Speed. Large numbers of people were so thoroughly tired of restrictions—and of not being able to open their stores to customers, travel to loved ones, or go to a movie or restaurant—that they rebelled against the many preventive measures put in place. The virus became entangled with political agendas, leading to various debates, decisions, and divisions. The first to emerge was the politics surrounding wearing masks; many people were tired of the rule to always wear a mask in public. Looking back, wearing a mask outdoors was inappropriate. Some felt that masks were a form of government control or an attempt to curtail people's freedom. Children were forced to mask even though the World Health Organization recommended against it.

The other major political controversy was surrounding the development and distribution of COVID vaccines. I recall initially many flocked to get the vaccine, and the elderly were prioritized. In Orange County, Florida, two women dressed as elderly grandmas to get the vaccine. Later, large numbers of Americans refused to get the vaccines for many reasons, such as the vaccines had not been tested long enough or had unknown side effects. There was also the distribution and prioritization of vaccines that only brought increased outrage among people.

The number of anti-maskers and anti-vaxxers increased, as did the politicization of preventative methods. To put it mildly, this was unfortunate. A virus doesn't recognize conservative or liberal, Republican or Democrat; it recognizes vulnerable lung cells. Show it some lung cells, and it doesn't ask if the person wore a mask on ninety-nine of the last one hundred days or doesn't like getting a shot; it attacks the lung cells. Boy, girl, billionaire, basketball star, ambulance driver, minister, bully, ninety-nine years old, or nine years old—it doesn't matter. It goes for the cells, and if there are inadequate antibodies or no natural immunity to ward off the attack, the virus multiplies inside the body and takes over millions of healthy cells.

My reporting and my comments are based on medical data and my direct hands-on patient care, no matter whether someone wants to hear that or not, Republican or Democrat. Due to the politicization of the virus, it was critical I provided accurate information. I was working on the front lines in the trenches, and I knew what was happening with COVID every day. Sometimes, misinformation undermined accurate reporting and further led to confusion. The conflicting narratives about the severity of the virus, the effectiveness of treatment, and appropriate response measures also added to the confusion. Despite all this, I felt obligated to give my viewers and my patients the most factual information surrounding COVID-19, the truth. I felt very strongly that viewers should hear the best and most recent data. I believed in speaking my truth and not bowing to political pressure on reporting, and in the end, it was effective.

John 8:32 ESV says, "And you will know the truth, and the truth will set you free."

Over time, the accumulated facts changed; we learned more. It was a dynamic, fluid situation. The more time elapsed, and the more data was collected, certain medicines or behaviors were demonstrated better—or worse—than had been thought before. All this was like on-the-job training. That is why we collect and examine data to see what is best and what is worse for increasing numbers of people. Consider, for example, the hydroxychloroquine prescription. There was some evidence for a short time that indicated hydroxychloroquine could help a certain percentage of patients. Governor Cuomo's office allowed its use in New York State. I prescribed it a few times myself. I recall some pharmacists laughing over the phone when I spoke to them about it. However, over time and with expanding data, hydroxychloroquine was shown to be ineffective. In other words, with increased usage and thus increased data, hydroxychloroquine was demonstrated to be not an effective general medicine for relieving the symptoms of

COVID-19, so we could no longer prescribe it. Other medicines should have been given a chance too. Meds are used off-label all the time. Viagra was created for babies' heart health and is now used secondarily for erectile dysfunction. How would we know if we didn't try? Lives could be saved, impotence could be treated, and perhaps relationships strengthened. Steroids, antidepressants, and antiparasitics were other meds tested for possible treatment.

We continued dealing with millions of data points from millions of people, all of whom were slightly different. Medical data largely deals in percentages, that is, percentages that are less than 100 percent. So, something can be good for 80 percent of the people but ineffective for the other 20 percent or downright harmful to 1 percent. In medicine, there usually are a lot of exceptions, so there is a lot of room for dissent for taking a position that goes against the majority or even the overwhelming majority. It has always been this way and always will be this way because everyone is slightly different. Physicians very often—some would say always—have to "play the odds." They have to say to patients, "This is what has worked for most people in your situation, and so it is likely to work for you. But there is a chance it might not." Physicians have to be honest with themselves, with the data that has been collected and presented, and with their patients. As a physician, I have sworn to do that, and I always will. Most doctors do.

When the politicization of COVID-19 began, many believed vaccines don't work and that masks don't work. Some say let mother nature have its way. We've been trying to prevent the virus from running wild, and despite these efforts, more than one million Americans have died of this disease. Instead, what we should have done was focused on the high-risk, most vulnerable groups and not clump everyone into a one-size-fits-all group. Around late 2020 and very early in 2021, when the first vaccines were becoming available and being made available only to the most vulnerable—that is, those over the age of seventy, healthcare workers, and workers in nursing homes—there was a kind of frenzy about getting the vaccines. People were rushing to have the injections; they lined up for hours. Some people were faking their age or their line of work just to get the shot. Where once our clinic was overwhelmed with COVID patients, now we were inundated with lines of people wanting the COVID vaccine.

Generally, vaccines are safe. They can have side effects. They boost a person's antibodies and help keep them out of the hospital. They did not stop the disease, but the more immunity in a community, the less the severity of disease. There is something called population herd immunity. The more people who have taken the vaccine, the lower the incidence of disease. When Bret Baier on Fox said to me, "The vaccines seem to be helping, but there is a lot of pushbacks," I said to him in return, "Yes, the vaccines cannot stop you from acquiring COVID but work by reducing symptoms and help to keep most people out of the hospital or dying." People needed the truth, which we later learned was that vaccines can only help reduce symptoms and lower the risk of serious suffering or death, and masks can help only if worn properly and consistently, otherwise, they are not effective as per the Cochrane Review, which is a review with multiple scientific studies and provides an unbiased analysis. I'll never forget my first patient who tested positive for COVID after being vaccinated. I was stunned. Her symptoms were mild.

Months into the pandemic, when the mask mandates issue came up, I was asked, "Who should wear masks?" As I've noted, medical data rarely indicates absolutes but rather percentages less than 100 percent, because not everyone has the same sex, age, weight, life experience, or same medical conditions and so forth.

If there might be—or have been—exceptions to a generalization you are about to make on television, then you have to admit that. Otherwise, it creates doubt. Trust is a critical aspect of a doctor-patient relationship. It leads to better outcomes and healthier, happier patients.

So, my reply about wearing masks was, "It depends on who you are and where you are. If you are in a community that has a high level of COVID-19 transmission and a massive outbreak of the disease, and you are not vaccinated, or you don't have natural immunity, and if you are elderly or have an underlying serious medical condition such as leukemia or breast cancer, lung disease, heart disease, obesity or diabetes, then you are at higher risk of serious illness if you contract COVID-19, and so wearing a well-fitted N95 mask in crowded public indoors is likely to do you a great deal of good." But, it should be a choice, and it should be noted they will only work with consistency. Doctors have to stick to science, to data that has been carefully collected and truthfully presented. It's the science that is going to help people, not wishful thinking, and not theories coming from people who don't have training in what organisms can do to cells in the human body.

Mandates are legal orders. It's better to lay facts in front of people, to educate them so that they see behaviors or remedies that they believe are not only good for themselves but for the community as well. Those who understand and accept science and act in accordance with facts might be the healthiest people and will do the most to help the community.

PRAYER

Dear Lord, we pray for all our political leaders. May you guide them in your wisdom and help them make the right choices when it comes to leadership. We pray for unity during our most difficult times; help us navigate our problems with compassion for one another. Please give us the strength and resilience to cope with all the challenges that come our way. Amen.

REFLECTION

The politicization of COVID only brought further division and confusion to a terrible situation. This was a time when people should have come together and treated each other with compassion and love, but at times, politics made some people treat each other with hatred, doubt, and unkindness. Instead of upholding the core values of Christian teachings, some people prioritized their partisan and personal interests. The COVID era reminds us of the importance of staying united. We should not pay mind to things that bring us disunity. Further, we should uphold measures that preserve the sanctity of life. If that means following health guidelines, then let it be so as a choice. After all, we are the land of the free and home of the brave.

THE BATTLE FOR CREDIBILITY AMID COVID-19 CHAOS

The delta variant arrived from India and was becoming a real problem. This was when politics had worked its way into how people thought about fighting the pandemic. Delta was really hitting school-aged children very hard, for one, because the vaccines hadn't been made available to their age group yet. So, I was asked, "Should kids be made to wear masks in school?" I said, "Global health organizations do not recommend it. Children spread this new variant more readily than the old variant, and because we are seeing thousands more children becoming infected, we need to remain vigilant in protecting the most vulnerable groups, which are the elderly and those with underlying medical conditions." The WHO does not recommend children wear masks, as it may interfere with social engagement, learning, and growth. Plus, children are low-risk for serious complications from COVID. My message on TV was, "Know your risks. Know what is going on around you and protect yourself."

As things began to be more and more political, it was important for me to avoid being political but rather to remain medical. I think I reached more people that way simply providing facts based on my experiences. My goal was to educate, to save lives. Some viewers thought, "Big pharma is paying you big bucks." The truth is, I have never been paid by big pharma to say anything. I stick to reporting what I see as a frontline physician and to statistics coming out of credible organizations. By the time of this writing, over the past few years, I've cared for and examined thousands of COVID-19-related patients. I know how they suffer. I know how people can modify their behaviors so that they reduce their chances of contracting the virus, or if they do contract the virus, how they can reduce the severity of the disease that they have. I am not a Republican; I am not a Democrat. I am a physician, and I am my own person. I don't say things to get ratings or stir people up. I speak facts to save lives.

I am not a TV doctor; I am a doctor who is on TV.

Unfortunately, there seems to have been a loss of confidence in authorities dealing with the pandemic. I think this is mainly because of the continually changing information, data, and conditions. The CDC makes recommendations. At one point, it was saying that if you were fully vaccinated, it was not necessary to wear masks indoors. Then they said that you should wear masks indoors even if you were fully vaccinated, but they made this change to their recommendation when the delta variant began to spread so rapidly across the country. The circumstances changed, and the CDC changed its recommendations as a result. But some people were confused by this and said they lost confidence in the CDC. It was a shame really. That trust needs to be rebuilt.

People also have to understand that there is various information but that the best information comes from people who have studied the problem for a long time or have been facing the problem on the front lines. Some government officials are well-meaning, but they run offices and manage people; they might be getting their information from field offices around the country. People feel more confident when they receive their information from the most well-informed sources and especially the caregivers and physicians who actually handle COVID-19 patients.

PRAYER

Lord, we pray that you always help us stand by the truth and make our voices heard. Whenever people want to silence our truth, may you speak for us. Please help us to always stand by our values and not be swayed by worldly things. Thank you for your goodness in our lives. Amen.

REFLECTION

In life, we will encounter people who try to silence you or disparage your faith. Many people in the Bible faced challenges when they tried to speak about the goodness of the Lord and His teachings. The Bible is full of stories of prophets, disciples, and believers who faced opposition while proclaiming the truth of God. Some were ostracized, jailed, abused, and persecuted for their beliefs. Even

Jesus himself met a lot of resistance to His teachings. Standing by your truth and defending your credibility as a Christian is how God wants you to be. If your information is from credible sources, you should remain steadfast in presenting accurate information, even when met with attempts to silence or discredit you. Credibility often shines brightest when surrounded by skepticism or doubt; your truth will eventually come to light.

CHAPTER 8

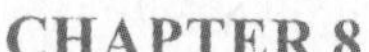

Compelling Courage: Empowering Your Health amid Vulnerability

> Effort and courage are not enough without patience and determination.
>
> —John F. Kennedy

By the time you read this book, I will have seen more than twenty thousand COVID-19-related patients. Some come into our healthcare facility afraid, barely having symptoms, and others come in for the first time when they are severely ill. It's important to note that some individuals may remain asymptomatic (showing no symptoms) but can still spread the virus to others. COVID-19 manifests in various states, and symptoms appear two to fourteen days after exposure to the virus; we have asymptomatic infections, mild-to-moderate, severe, and critical symptoms. Individuals with asymptomatic infections may never necessarily develop any symptoms; if they do, they are often mild symptoms that go unnoticed. This issue makes the situation tricky and a bit dangerous because even those with asymptomatic infections can still spread the virus without knowing they have it. Mild-to-moderate symptoms are characterized by fever, cough, fatigue, headache, sore throat, and loss of taste or smell (anosmia). They also experience gastrointestinal symptoms such as diarrhea and vomiting. Individuals with mild-to-moderate symptoms often do not need to be hospitalized; they can recover at home with rest, hydration, and over-the-counter medications to manage symptoms. Patients with severe cases can experience acute respiratory distress syndrome (ARDS), characterized by severe shortness of breath, rapid breathing, low blood oxygen levels, and lung infiltrates visible on imaging scans. They may have chest pains or feel a lot of pressure in their chest and have a high fever of above 101°F or 38°C. Their face or lips may turn blue or grayish due to oxygen deprivation. Severe cases require hospitalization for oxygen therapy and supportive care—these cannot be managed at home. Some may need to be on ventilators.

The worst state is when a patient advances to the critical stage. This is when severe cases deteriorate further, and patients experience multi-organ failure and can go into septic shock. Other symptoms may include confusion, bluish lips or face, severe chest pain, and an inability to stay awake. These patients need close monitoring and should be admitted to the intensive care unit and put on mechanical ventilation.

As a medical doctor working full-time during the COVID-19 pandemic, I saw my fair share of the ravages of COVID. No medical training could have prepared me for the relentless onslaught of patients during the peak of the COVID pandemic; I saw so many patients daily—each seemingly sicker than the last. One evening, during a long, fourteen-hour shift, I went to check on a patient who had just been brought into the facility. She was an older woman struggling to breathe. Her eyes were wide with fear, and her oxygen levels were dangerously low. I could hear the rasping sound of her labored breaths, a sound that had become all too familiar. I quickly connected her to oxygen and administered medications, but her condition remained critical. She desperately needed mechanical ventilation, so we transferred her to the intensive care unit. Her son, who had brought her in, was beside himself with worry, and we were forced to send him away because we couldn't have more people at the hospital who did not have to be there. It broke my heart to see him break down and cry so much; he didn't want to leave. He even asked if he could stay outside the gate. I assured him, "I understand how worried you must be about your mother. We're doing everything we can to provide the best care possible."

"I appreciate all your efforts, doctors, but I can't leave her alone in the hospital. Please let me stay around. I will feel so guilty leaving her here alone. I promise not to interfere with anyone, please," he pleaded.

"I completely understand your concern, but she won't be alone. We have a team of doctors and nurses working around the clock to help her recover quickly." We were already overflowing with patients, and we couldn't have more people contributing to the growing crowd. I did not force him to leave. I could not break families apart.

"Okay, doctor, I guess at this point, all I can do is pray for her and hope she beats the virus," he said. I was pleased to know he was Christian and looked to God in times of need.

"Go home and take better care of yourself too, and as you pray, ask the Lord to renew your strength. Remember that the Lord is with you through this trying period. He says so in Isaiah 41:13 NIV, "For I am the Lord your God who takes hold of your right hand and says to you, 'Do not fear; I will help you.'"

"Thank you, doctor. Your words provide a sense of peace in the midst of all this," he said before eventually heading home that night.

But the never-ending horror show continued—till now I have visions of black body bags and semitrucks used as morgues. A middle-aged woman was coughing violently in the next bed. Each cough seemed to wrack her whole body, and her face contorted in pain. I checked her oxygen levels and noticed that they were dropping rapidly. The fear etched in the woman's eyes mirrored that of the nurses who had been attending to her. I quickly administered supplemental oxygen through a high-flow nasal cannula. This action was in a bid to increase the concentration of oxygen in the patient's blood. I then ordered our nurses to monitor the patient's vital signs, including oxygen saturation levels, heart rate, blood pressure, and respiratory rate. Then, I would assess the progress later to determine the next best course of action. For some patients, their diaphragm muscles would tire out, and they would need help breathing.

I encountered cases of people struggling with the virus, from young adults gasping for air to people on ventilators with unrecognizable faces due to the swelling. Some days were really difficult, and my heart grew heavier with each passing hour. If it were not for the support of family and the word of God that comforted me during these difficult moments, I would have lost my mind. I will never forget how God held me together; 2 Corinthians 1:3–4 NIV says: "Praise be to the God and Father of our Lord Jesus Christ, the Father of compassion and the God of all comfort, who comforts us in all our troubles so that we can comfort those in any trouble with the comfort we ourselves receive from God."

When it comes to staying healthy, keep yourself safe and take care of the people around you. Taking good care of our bodies is also maintaining stewardship of the Temple of God; 1 Corinthians 6:19–20 NIV teaches us that our bodies are the Temple of God:

> Do you not know that your bodies are
> temples of the Holy Spirit, who is in you,
> whom you have received from God? You are
> not your own; you were bought at a price.
> Therefore, honor God with your bodies.

So, by preventing our bodies from harm, we are also taking care of the Temple of God.

PRAYER

Father Lord, we come before you with grateful hearts, recognizing that you are God above all. We pray that in the face of challenges such as COVID-19, you may give us guidance and strength to make wise decisions that honor you and protect the well-being of ourselves and others. Grant us the humility to follow the guidance of health experts and adhere to hygiene recommendations. Let our actions testify to our faith, showing the world that we are united in love and care for one another.

REFLECTION

In this chapter, we will reflect on our duties and obligations to ourselves and others. As a doctor, I believe that taking preventive measures to protect ourselves and others from any illness is a responsible act and a reflection of our love and care for our neighbor. The Bible teaches us to prioritize the well-being of those around us, and there has never been a better time to practice this principle than during a pandemic. In Proverbs 22:3, God calls us to be wise stewards of our resources, including our health and the healthcare system's resources. If the infected worry about the uninfected and take precautions, it may help reduce spread. How do you practice caring for the vulnerable? We protect the weak, embodying the principle of looking out for "the least of these" as outlined in Matthew 25:40. We are also taught to honor authority. Following the pandemic, there were public health guidelines that were outlined by the authorities to guide us. Rules and guidelines are necessary because otherwise, there would be no order. At times however, the guidelines were outdated and did not "follow the science."

THE PLIGHT OF VULNERABLE POPULATIONS DURING THE PANDEMIC

If COVID's effect was sometimes hard on healthy, young adults, it makes you wonder how it affected the most vulnerable populations. The most vulnerable people in a pandemic are those at a higher risk of severe illness or complications if they contract a disease. Many factors can make someone susceptible to the COVID-19 virus, such as age, underlying health conditions, living situations, and limited access to health care. It is essential to also look at how the pandemic affected these groups of people. Now, let us look at different groups of vulnerable populations affected by COVID-19.

Obesity

By far, the most troubling cases I have seen over these years have been of people who are obese. These people are most vulnerable to severe cases, hospitalizations, and death. The extra weight makes it more difficult to breathe.

Of course, obesity carries with it conditions that are unhealthy. Obese patients are much more likely to suffer from diabetes, heart disease, hypertension, and stress. These are severe health conditions in themselves, but they also contribute to a diminished capacity of the immune system to fight off viral infections, of which COVID is very serious. Why? Because extra adipose tissue (fat) leads to inflammation in the body. In addition, when the COVID virus infects the respiratory system of obese people, they have more incredible difficulty than thinner people, merely expanding and contracting the lungs to absorb sufficient oxygen into the bloodstream.

Treating obese patients can be more challenging due to the difficulty of administering medications, obtaining imaging, and performing intubations or other medical procedures. Without completing a medical procedure and getting to the underlying issue, it is often difficult to treat the problem. Most obese patients also did not want to subject themselves to the torturous examinations, so they opted to stay home. Obese patients also unintentionally strain healthcare resources; they often have complex medical needs due to multiple comorbidities such as diabetes, heart disease, and respiratory conditions. Healthcare providers must allocate more time and resources to manage these conditions effectively. Additionally, obese patients who develop severe respiratory distress due to COVID may require advanced ventilator support, which can be more challenging in individuals with excess body weight. Specialized equipment and adjustments are often necessary to accommodate their needs, and not many hospitals can afford them. But nonetheless, it is our duty to care for all patients regardless of size.

There is a theory that obesity can influence the effectiveness of vaccines. Some studies suggest that obese individuals may have a reduced immune response to vaccines, including those for COVID, which could make them more susceptible to complications. Being obese indeed presents more challenges, especially when fighting off additional diseases and infections. From what I have seen in my patients, a thin sixty-year-old person with heart disease will have less trouble with COVID than a forty-year-old with no medical problems other than morbid obesity.

It is essential to take care of our bodies. At the same time, the Bible does not necessarily mention obesity, but it underscores the importance of caring for our bodies, living in a way that pleases God, and avoiding excesses. Proverbs 23:20–21 NIV says: "Do not join those who drink too much wine or gorge themselves on meat, for drunkards and gluttons become poor, and drowsiness clothes them in rags."

And also, in 1 Corinthians 10:31 NIV: "So, whether you eat or drink or whatever you do, do it all for the glory of God."

Children

Children are another special class. When COVID began to spread in 2020, the common thinking was that children were less vulnerable. Generally, this is true, in part because COVID enters our cells through ACE receptors. The density of these receptors in our lungs may be less in children, potentially influencing the severity of infection. Reports indicated that children were not contracting the disease at the same rate as adults. Some thought this was because children had immune systems that could better fight off the SARS-CoV-2 virus. More likely, children had lower infection rates than adults because it was adults who were catching the disease and then spreading it to other adults during adult activities, namely spreading the virus at their places of work, at bars and restaurants, sporting events, and so on. Moreover, during the early months of the pandemic, most of the focus was on nursing homes or assisted living places because the virus was spreading rapidly, and the disease was the most fatal among the elderly.

Children were less vulnerable and less infected initially. Keen observers might have predicted this would change once family members brought the virus into their homes, and both students and teachers spread it into schools. Naturally, children did begin to get sick in large numbers. The fact that they were hospitalized at lower rates than people in higher age brackets again suggested that children could fight the virus better and that attention should focus more on older persons, not the youngest.

Children can be vulnerable to viral infections and susceptible to severe consequences, but fortunately, this is quite rare. Children have smaller airways than grown-ups. Inflammations in these airways can come close to constricting the airways entirely, or secretions can more readily and swiftly clog them up.

Most children with the virus were asymptomatic or had mild symptoms. They might experience symptoms similar to a cold or mild flu, such as fever, cough, and fatigue, making it challenging to identify cases and control transmission. They can, therefore, still spread the virus to others, including more vulnerable adults. It's estimated by the CDC that most children had already contracted COVID. This leads to natural immunity, although not everlasting.

Consequently, any viral infection in children or adults can be severe, and the medics must watch them carefully if they have an underlying medical condition like cystic fibrosis or leukemia.

Other Comorbidities

Severe underlying conditions, or comorbidities, as we refer to them, also increase the susceptibility to severe illness. People with cancer, AIDS, hypertension, atrial fibrillation (irregular heartbeat), high cholesterol, afflictions of the immune system, or who are taking medications that compromise the immune system are also more vulnerable than most to harsh cases of disease. When they impact the body's ability to fight off the virus, it increases the risks of severe complications. Cardiovascular diseases affect the respiratory system and can strain the cardiovascular system. People with diabetes will experience more severe symptoms due to potentially compromised immune response and inflammation. Other chronic respiratory diseases increase the risk of respiratory distress from COVID.

Kidney diseases weaken the body's immunity, which can hinder the body's ability to fight off infections like chemotherapy treatments for cancer. People with these and many other comorbidities are at a high risk of developing severe complications. These people need special care and should be in continuous touch with their doctor.

Marginalized Communities

The coronavirus has not hit communities across the country equally. The upper class and upper-middle class have been less affected. Why? Probably because they are healthier to begin with and have the money to have good health insurance and money to use healthcare providers over and above what their insurance companies pay for.

But lower-income people tend not to have the best diets, often work in conditions that wear down their health, get less sleep, have either no health insurance or insurance plans that provide less coverage and require higher deductibles for treatment, and, because of less coverage of benefits, tend to avoid going to healthcare facilities on account of lacking the means to pay for services or copays.

In my experience with the pandemic, the Hispanic community, especially immigrants and non-English speakers, has been hit hardest. Many have high blood pressure, diabetes, or stressful lives, which beat down the immune system. I was once helping care for patients in Corona, New York. I recall taking care of an obese Hispanic man with new onset diabetes with COVID who needed to be hospitalized. He was homeless, he didn't speak English, he had COVID pneumonia, he didn't know he had diabetes, and his blood sugar was over five hundred. He barely survived.

People in immigrant communities also tend to seek care late. If they lack legal status in the United States, they may fear discovery and deportation. Even if they are confident of their status, they often don't know where to go, how they will communicate with whomever they will see, or fear that they will contract another and worse disease in the emergency room or healthcare facility they walk into. People from marginalized communities also have limited internet access; this results in limited access to accurate health information and updates about the pandemic, affecting the ability to make informed decisions.

Another reason that holds them back is fear that their family will not be able to visit them. Things are better now than they were four years ago, but it is so sad to see someone very ill, on the verge of death or dying, and having the fear that they will die alone or without seeing the people who love them and instead must settle on being surrounded by strangers in medical gear. These people who come in late—a week or two weeks after they suffer symptoms—often have very low oxygen levels. Hospitals have to decide whether or not to put them on ventilators, which can be more dire than merely supplying oxygen through nostril tubes. Higher rates of poverty, crowded living conditions, and limited access to health care contributed to increased COVID deaths or complications for some communities. Preexisting health conditions made it much more difficult.

THE UNSEEN SAFETY AND HEALTH STRUGGLES OF UNDOCUMENTED IMMIGRANTS

Imagine a significant number of people living in a particular community choosing not to report being beaten, burglarized, or raped. Law enforcement would work tirelessly to get solutions to the safety issue.

This scenario is playing out in my town and across the country as we see the erosion of the immigration process—it is an issue that's staining the sanctity of our justice system. A recent survey showed that 78 percent of domestic and sexual violence victims who are immigrants have concerns about seeking help from the police[1].

"...I DON'T HAVE PAPERS, AND I CAN'T GO BACK TO MY COUNTRY..."

In the heart of every city, some stories echo the human spirit's resilience. These are the stories of immigrants who continue to fight for their lives with dignity despite their fear of deportation. This is both humbling and inspiring.

One such story is of a patient I met on 57th Street. He was a man with a knife wound in his stomach. He had been stabbed and suffered an injury severe enough to necessitate immediate emergency care. Yet, he had not called the police or sought help from a hospital.

---

1 National Network to End Domestic Violence. "Survey Reveals Impact of Increased Immigration Enforcement on Victims Experiencing Domestic Violence and Sexual Assault." National Network to End Domestic Violence, May 18, 2017. https://nnedv.org/latest_update/increased-immigration-enforcement/.

But why? The answer tore me apart, and I couldn't hold my tears: "I don't have papers, and I can't go back to my country." His fear was so profound that he chose to risk his life rather than face the possibility of survival in his homeland after deportation. His courage in the face of such a health emergency moved me deeply. Securing our borders could have prevented his injury. But we have wide-open borders, people from all over the world entering illegally.

Then there was the tragic case of a young teenage patient I had on 42nd Street, raped by another illegal immigrant. Another patient I cared for, a young boy, came in writhing in abdominal pain and was rushed to the surgeon for suspected appendicitis. There were similar stories, and each story is proof of the struggles faced by these children. Yet, despite the need for emergency care, these people didn't dial 911 for fear of deportation and continue to illegally cross our southern border despite deadly risk for themselves and their children.

I remember a heart-wrenching incident at the Northwest Hospital ICU in Springdale. A young immigrant, ravaged by AIDS, was on the brink of death. He had persistent uncontrollable diarrhea, a severe rash, and organ failure. His mother, in another country, was denied the chance to be with her son in his final moments. Yet we have open southern borders with thousands entering daily.

Then there are sad stories of immigrants meeting horrific ends. For instance, fifty people suffocated in the back of a semitruck driven by an intoxicated drunken driver high on meth who left them all to roast to death in the summer heat. Then there are immigrants and soldiers trying to save them drowning in rivers or falling prey to human trafficking and sexual exploitation.

IT'S SAD

For most undocumented immigrants experiencing domestic and sexual violence, the threat of possible deportation is compounded by exposing their undocumented status. They are also afraid of being separated from their loved ones. When the community and law enforcement are overloaded with open borders, an opportunity to stop current and future violence against men, women, and children is missed.

In fact, the policies that blur the line between the community law enforcement and immigration processes endanger the safety of undocumented immigrants and American citizens. The victims' access to justice is, in fact, partly blocked by the same people whose duty is to protect them and fight for their justice, but they can't because they are overwhelmed with administrative tasks.

A BETTER OPTION

Amid all this chaos and tragedy, there's a beacon of hope: legal immigration. My parents and grandparents, for instance, legally immigrated to the USA through Ellis Island in NYC. Immigrants undergo a series of tests as well as vaccinations and background checks to ensure they pose no health or security risks. Deuteronomy 24:14 warns us against taking advantage of others, especially foreigners residing in our towns. So, how about we implement immigration policies that protect human rights and the safety of our nation?

PRAYER

Dear heavenly Father, you are a God of justice and love, and we lift up those often overlooked and underserved. We pray for your grace, mercy, and provision to shine upon them. Father, we ask you to protect children vulnerable to exploitation, abuse, and neglect. We also pray for every other group of people who are most susceptible to risks. May you help them overcome the challenges that are brought by the condition they are in. Amen.

REFLECTION

The plight of marginalized populations, especially during economic turmoil or war, calls us to respond with compassion, empathy, and a commitment to justice. There are often many disparities in life, from society to the judicial system and even the healthcare system. The teachings of Jesus remind us of the significance of reaching out to those who are often overlooked, especially during a health crisis or natural disaster. Every person, regardless of their social status, ethnicity, or economic situation, is created in the image of God and bears inherent dignity and worth. Jesus consistently demonstrated compassion and empathy towards marginalized individuals. He embraced the outcast, healed the sick, and offered hope to those who felt forgotten. As followers of Christ, we're called to extend a hand of compassion to those who are suffering most during this crisis. The marginalized populations are often overlooked when it comes to being given a service. Jesus's life was a servanthood model; He washed His disciples' feet, humbling Himself to serve those seemingly beneath Him. We should all embody this kind of humility when dealing with others.

Ignorance and Naysayers

"It won't happen to me." Over one million Americans have died of COVID-19 (as of December 2023). Many of them thought they would not catch the disease for one reason or another, such as they did not live in assisted living facilities, they did not live in cities, they were healthy, they were young, and so on. The problem is that COVID is a virus that attaches itself to human respiratory cells wherever it can find them, no matter where the host lives, no matter his or her race, no matter his or her political leanings, no matter his or her wealth, job, country, or age. The virus is an equal opportunity threat; all it cares about is respiratory system cell walls—if they are of the right kind, it will pierce the cell walls, infect them, and make their hosts sick.

"I won't take the vaccine because…" There are various ways naysayers end this sentence: "…it won't work," "…it will harm me," "…it is part of government control," "…it was rushed into production and not properly proven safe." The Trump administration's Operation Warp Speed was a great accomplishment that from my experience saved many lives and prevented many hospitalizations, especially among the elderly and vulnerable groups.

"I might as well catch the virus, suffer through a mild case, and become immune that way." There is some truth to this, but you can become infected and then spread the virus to others before you have symptoms and know you are sick. Sure, you could catch the virus at your place of work and then give it to your children or grandparents without you even knowing it. For another, you are only guessing you will have a mild case. There is no guarantee that you will. Most will have a mild case. There is the threat of what is often called "long COVID." This is the variety of medical discomfort from which many people suffer months or even years after the initial infection and after the worst of the disease has faded from their bodies. Long COVID is poorly understood because there has been too little time to study it. However, the SARS-CoV-2 virus in some people seems to cause more than mere short-term damage to the respiratory system; it can leave lasting damage to the lungs. In addition, some people who recovered from COVID and seem otherwise healthy have suffered micro blood clots, heart inflammation, lingering fatigue, brain fog, shortness of breath, and inability to concentrate. It is foolish to take the position that there is a benefit to catching COVID. There isn't. After recovering from COVID, you will have natural immunity that protects you for a short period of time. I have had patients catch COVID several times.

Fortunately, we now have vaccines that minimize the dangers of COVID. Vaccinated and unvaccinated can still become infected, but as of now, the vaccinated are less likely to become seriously ill, be hospitalized, be intubated, or die of the disease. They are far less likely to pass the virus on to their friends, relatives, and loved ones. If they do get sick, they are less likely to suffer the troubles of long COVID. Usually, vaccinated people are less likely to be hospitalized.

You might wonder how I deal with those reluctant to get the COVID vaccine. First, I don't try to assume the role of a superior being vax pusher. I explain to patients who come in that we do not have the vaccine in, so we are not about to strong-arm anyone into having an injection during their visit. I explain the ingredients in the vaccines, the research and results provided to us, the fact that the vaccines were developed and tested on thousands, have been given to millions worldwide, and that there is a possibility of adverse reactions as is with any vaccine. Polio, hepatitis, measles, mumps, rubella, and tetanus vaccines are exceptional in protecting our health and preventing serious debilitating disease. The COVID vaccine can only help minimize symptoms; it cannot prevent disease like we were initially told.

I try as best I can to tell them that I will only provide information, and I do not have stock in the company or get kickbacks. I ask them about their questions and concerns, and I explain the differences among the vaccines. I say Moderna is the strongest, Pfizer is in the middle, and Johnson & Johnson is the least strong—so if they fear a reaction or side effect, they might choose the weakest one or none at all. I explain that the FDA has approved all three; this may change in the future based on new information. I tell them they can talk to their doctors and their pharmacists and come back if they have further questions. My job is only to provide information, and it is their choice if they choose to be vaccinated or not. After all, this is America—land of the free.

I feel that if you give calm and reasonable education and are not judgmental, your words begin to sink in and have a good effect.

I do the same when I talk with parents about giving hepatitis shots to their children. I don't get argumentative or pushy, but I provide sound medical information. Parents usually come around to the right choice for their children when they have gone home and thought it over.

What I have outlined I also use with other sorts of health choices. It's concerning that some people are making unhealthy choices, but we doctors have to be patient and keep gently educating them. We talk to smokers about the ill effects of smoking while suggesting ways they can begin to quit. We have to keep doing this at every visit because when people hear it enough, it begins to sink in, and one day our words may work.

We must patiently keep at it: educate, encourage, and talk about the benefits of eating healthy, exercising regularly, getting plenty of sleep, and not using drugs or drinking excessively.

Communication, believe it or not, is a big part of medicine, of keeping people healthy and getting them back to health if they are unhealthy. This is why I take pride in reporting accurate and up-to-date health information as a TV medical contributor, hoping my information will reach as many people as possible and help direct them to get the best health care. I receive hundreds of emails, letters, and phone calls of gratitude for providing information in an easy-to-understand manner, so I think it's working. It's an honor and privilege to teach and to serve God by caring for others.

NURTURING WELLNESS AFTER A POSITIVE COVID-19 TEST

If you ever test positive on a home test, don't panic. Settle down and begin to treat your symptoms with the notion—and the hope—that you will have a mild case, as is true of most people who catch a virus. Stay home and rest, drink some hot tea with honey, take some BC BOOST—vitamin C, zinc, and vitamin D3. Take some vitamin B12 if you feel fatigue. Stay home so you do not spread the virus to loved ones or get sicker. Most people don't need to go to a healthcare facility or a medical office unless you have trouble breathing, have chest pain, or feel weak or lethargic. If you have mild symptoms and test positive at home, you don't need to go to your doctor for a confirmation test. Assume you have it and act appropriately. Going into a healthcare facility "to confirm" a test result only jams up the facility's waiting room, takes up doctors' or nurses' time, and exposes everyone in the facility to the virus you are carrying. If you are elderly or have an underlying medical condition, then that's a different story—you may need treatment, so call your doctor. The old fourteen-day quarantine is now gone.

As a Christian, this is the best time to turn to God and make it right with Him. Turn to prayer for healing and restoration. Ask for God's guidance and strength as you navigate this challenging time. Trust that God's love and presence are with you, providing comfort and hope. You should also seek solace in the word of God; spend time studying the Bible and reflecting on its teachings. Psalm 46:1 KJV says, "God is our refuge and strength, an ever-present help in trouble."

The Lord Father reassures us that we will never be alone, even in our weaknesses; He will always be our strength. Once again, Isaiah 41:10 NIV reminds us, "So do not fear, for I am with you; do not be dismayed, for I am your God. I will strengthen you and help you; I will uphold you with my righteous right hand."

It is also essential to have a positive mindset through times like this. Adding stress to a complicated situation will only worsen your condition; embrace a positive attitude rooted in faith. Romans 8:28 NIV says, "And we know that in all things God works for the good of those who love him," and Philippians 4:13 NKJV also reminds us, "I can do all things through Christ who strengthens me."

PRAYER

Almighty and ever-loving Father, we come before you with heavy hearts, mourning the pain and suffering of all who have been infected and affected by disease. The pandemic has ended, but it has brought many illnesses, loss, fear, and uncertainty; many families have lost their loved ones. We seek your presence, comfort, and healing for all impacted. May your healing hand restore the health of those still yet to fully recover from the virus-related complications.

REFLECTION

Trials and tribulations sometimes come as a test of your faith. Reflecting on your relationship with God is crucial during difficult times. In the case of COVID, or any disease, as a Christian, you should prioritize both your physical health and your spiritual well-being.

While facing uncertainty, lean on your faith in God's plan. Trust that He is in control and has a purpose for you, even under challenging circumstances. While relying on prayer and spiritual strength, it's equally important to follow evidence-based medical advice and public health guidelines to ensure your overall well-being.

Also, thank God; this may be very difficult to do, especially when you're going through a very tough period, but the truth is God's grace and mercy never leaves you at any point. Offer thanks to God for healing and recovery during and after any illness.

SMALL STEPS, BIG RESULTS: WHAT PEOPLE CAN DO TO CRUSH THE PANDEMIC

Every time there is a new infection, there is a human failing. I don't think this has been emphasized enough. The pandemic is a *human problem*. The pandemic is not a hurricane, twelve inches of rain in twelve hours, or a string of tornados. We cannot do anything about those things except to do our best to prepare for them when they come. By contrast, the COVID problem is a result of human behavior. True, a virus is a natural protein construct, unless it was consciously manipulated in a lab like COVID-19. Still, every transmission from one person to another has been due to a human error. Someone did not cough into his elbow, went out in public when sick, went to a gathering where people were infected, did not wash hands, or simply didn't know they had COVID, and so on. If, for two weeks, no transmission of the COVID virus took place from one person to another, the pandemic would be over—we tried that, but it didn't work. Remember fifteen days to slow the spread?

What can people do? Simply, keep yourself in the best health possible at baseline. Stay active, maintain a healthy weight, and eat nutritious foods; avoid processed food loaded with chemicals. Follow instructions and adhere to the normal standard common-sense health precautions. Stay informed, be prepared to adapt to changing circumstances, and follow updated guidance as the situation evolves—health and medicine are dynamic.

Remember, this is not a hurricane or other natural disaster. Humans made this pandemic, and humans can unmake it.

PRAYER

Dear Lord, we ask you for strength to persevere through any illness or pandemic, to support one another, and to stand firm against any disease.

REFLECTION

As individuals and communities, we are often faced with unprecedented challenges that need our collective efforts to overcome. A crisis like COVID was a global pandemic that affected us all; through our shared determination, we overcame it. As we reflect on this journey, we are reminded of our capacity to adapt, to care for one another, and to make sacrifices for the greater good. Sometimes change is needed—if we follow through with necessary changes, then success is imminent. We would have to embrace new ways of working, learning, and connecting and adapt to a rapidly changing world. This makes us stronger. We are a resilient nation.

FRONTLINE HEROES: WHAT THE MEDICAL PROFESSION CAN DO TO CRUSH THE PANDEMIC

Doctors play one of the most crucial roles in crushing a pandemic, yet they often do not get appreciated enough.

First, we need more doctors and nurses. At present, we don't have enough to work with the millions of people who have had, have, or are about to have COVID or any other type of disease. COVID significantly underscored the shortage of doctors and nurses in hospitals worldwide. The number of medical professionals could not contain the overflowing number of patients that flooded hospitals nationwide. Many doctors had to work long shifts to see more patients.

The medical profession, the public, and the media must stand behind doctors and nurses who are on the front lines of a pandemic. Doctors and nurses are quitting their jobs at unsettling rates. They were overworked during the pandemic. They are stressed out. They are discouraged. They get burned out, and they quit. People must be mindful that medical staff need time off, quality time with their families, sleep, and vacations. Doctors and dentists have the highest rates of suicide because of the stress their occupations put them under.

Doctors, by law, must report specific incidents of disease. For example, when they see a case of gonorrhea or tuberculosis, they must report it to the local public health department. This is not government spying or depriving people of rights. Long ago, people understood that infectious diseases could be stopped in a community when cases were first detected and proper measures taken. Remember the old expression, "A stitch in time saves nine"?

If a community understands a disease has appeared in its midst, it can warn everyone, treat those exposed or isolate the cases, and order preventative medicines so that the disease is localized and defeated before becoming a widespread menace. But that can only happen if the community—through the public health department—knows about it.

Doctors were once required to report to health officials when they diagnosed a patient with COVID. They were not allowed to fly on an airplane or travel on a train or bus unless they had proof of a negative test. At the beginning of the pandemic, COVID spread almost to everyone on a plane carrying passengers and on massive cruise ships. I recall being live on TV for breaking news, on set with Dana Perino, talking to a cruise ship passenger aboard the Princess Cruise who was stuck on the ship in California. She was not allowed to depart the ship due to fear of COVID spread because more than six hundred passengers tested positive for COVID—yet she was in desperate need of her medication that she had already gone days without, but she had to wait as health officials were scrambling on what to do for the infected passengers; the ship circled for days until it docked. In the meantime, I reassured the patient that we would do everything to get her her meds immediately.

Doctors can educate the public about the virus, prevention measures, and vaccine safety, combating misinformation. As I mentioned earlier, I took it upon myself to teach the public about COVID-19, and it was a blessing to have the platform to get the facts out there. I provided patients and viewers with the most correct and up-to-date information, which helped them in many ways to prevent contracting the virus, and informed them of the proper measures to take to keep themselves safe and what to do if they tested positive. Medical professionals can also contribute to scientific research, clinical trials, and the development of new treatments and vaccines. Through the efforts of medical professionals, we were able to get vaccines that helped to reduce the rate of death and hospitalizations.

The medical community should advocate for public health measures based on scientific evidence. They can also engage with communities to build trust and promote adherence to health guidelines. Many people fail to follow health guidelines because they have lost faith in the healthcare system. Medical professionals need to rebuild trust in their communities to serve them better.

Additionally, doctors handle a lot of patients; they must protect themselves so that they can prevent transmitting disease to other patients and picking up infections as well. Doctors should always wear the proper protective gear and ensure their safety by wearing appropriate personal protective equipment (PPE) in addition to handwashing, the best way to prevent the spread of most diseases.

Look over the horizon. The medical community has to pay attention not just to the present but to the future. We must prepare for the possibility of new variants and ensure government and pharmaceutical companies update and modify tests accordingly that can detect new variants and treat them when they occur. The medical community cannot be complacent by thinking it now has all the tools and test kits it needs; new variants will make the manufacture of new test kits necessary as well as new treatments. We must be two steps ahead, especially while gain of function and risky research is still ongoing throughout the world. We don't know what the next disease X will entail, so the best defense is preparation, not procrastination.

LEADING THE CHARGE: WHAT GOVERNMENT CAN DO TO CRUSH THE PANDEMIC

The years of the pandemic have been learning years, like "on-the-job training" for the government, meaning all levels of government—federal, state, county, city—and not just the politicians who control those governments but also the agencies that operate within those governments. They were confronted with a situation they had never expected. They thought that the pandemic of 1918–1920 was ancient history. So when our twenty-first-century pandemic hit, nearly all the politicians, governments, and agencies were caught unprepared and unaware. That means they had to formulate remedies as they went along. That didn't work out very well.

For one thing, governments tended to respond to the growing pandemic of late winter and early spring of 2020 in absolute terms. They shouldn't have been so absolute, such as saying, "You have to wear masks." They should have determined for whom and where and when masks were appropriate, for example, only indoors or in communities where the infection rate was high. Being more conditional rather than being so absolute would have saved more of the economy from shutting down and businesses going from good times to zero customers in a week. It was a shock too much to bear for the service industries, the travel industry, airlines, a lot of retail, and so on. Almost immediately, because of people staying home, the streets were deserted, the shopping malls empty, and the restaurants without diners. The main problem early on was in our nursing homes and assisted living facilities. Here is where we should have concentrated our efforts to protect the residents and the staff, to stop the virus in these places, and to thwart the spread of the disease to the larger community beyond.

To this day, I think some of the mandates and cautions were too severe and worked too much against getting the economy back to normal.

Our federal government and federal agencies should have paid more attention to what was happening in China, especially in 2019, and pressed the Chinese harder to give us information on the genetic makeup of the virus they were admitting to having trouble with. They were more focused on trying to impeach the president rather than keep Americans safe.

I think the government has to lighten up on mandates. N95s can help, especially in indoor situations where people might cough, sneeze, or vigorously exhale. But having to wear masks all the time and as the pandemic winds down? I don't think so. I was seeing children with abscesses behind their ears where the elastic bands were rubbing their skin and rashes on their faces where the masks were. I had to wear an N95 at work for long hours, for thirteen- to fourteen-hour shifts; it's very hard to breathe. Let's just use common sense.

Governments should have concentrated on the most vulnerable—the older people and people with preexisting illnesses—and let other people carry on a more normal life, let them keep the economy on track. Severe lockdowns caused harm in different ways too. People could not go in for regular checkups, mammograms, heart screenings, skin biopsies, colonoscopies; tooth decay persisted, blood sugar levels rose, and so forth. Many did not exercise. General healthiness declined. People gained weight. Children did not get their regular childhood vaccines for measles, mumps, rubella, polio, and more—and not just in the United States but worldwide, which puts us in danger even in our country. This is why now we have measles outbreaks and TB outbreaks.

Here was another overreaction: requiring children under five to be vaccinated to attend school. Leave them alone. We can crush this pandemic without vaccinating toddlers who have natural immunity. Nobody should have been mandated to vaccinate. It should be a choice. My heart breaks for soldiers, marines, airmen, firefighters, and police officers who lost their jobs for standing up for their right to say no.

The federal government and federal agencies were not prepared for a pandemic, one that would sweep the country within weeks. We had to resort to tents and hospital ships. Morgues were not ready; bodies had to be stored in refrigerated trucks.

And the preparedness problem persisted. The governments and government agencies were not prepared for the delta variant. They thought the pandemic was petering out. Then, the delta variant struck in the summer of 2021. When the delta infection rates were declining, the government and agencies were not prepared for what came next—the omicron variant. In the United States, omicron steamrolled in soon after Thanksgiving. Daily cases reached almost four times higher than the highest previous levels under the delta variant or the original configuration of 2020, with more than 750,000 new cases daily. It was astonishing. The lines of patients out the door were miles long.

Another problem was making predictions and proclamations that confused the public. Wear masks, don't wear masks, and so on. People became confused, and they were already anxious. Some became angry. I think a lot of the anti-vaxxer movement sprang from people who heard the government pronouncements but found them not logical or helpful; this led them to conclude that any government recommendation was suspect, if not downright wrong.

So, what did the government do right? Well, one thing it did right in 2020 was launch Operation Warp Speed. This was the development of the vaccines, which were desperately needed and were developed in record time. The government cut through red tape and other obstacles to get the vaccines made and out to the public in a period never attempted or achieved before. The government let the pharmaceutical companies develop the vaccines in record time without what otherwise would have been years of study and testing. These vaccines saved huge numbers of people. The government also allowed some treatments such as hydroxychloroquine, which was not a valid medicine for everyone but did some good for some people until it was removed as a treatment. Eventually, they used remdesivir, vitamin C, and steroids.

We need governments to work so that people don't have to wait three hours to be tested. We need the federal government to use the Defense Production Act to spur the manufacture of equipment that will help put a pandemic under control when needed. We must stockpile equipment, PPE, masks, tests, and medicines for new variants or disease X.

Governments should not have kept children out of schools for as long as they did. Children are the lowest risks when it comes to COVID. Many children needed to be in school to get the meals and nutrition they were used to previously and were not receiving at home. It is also in schools that students can receive counseling and mental health resources. Sadly, for some children, being at school was a safe haven away from abuse and neglect at home. At home all of the time, children's anxiety levels rose, and their mental health deteriorated. Suicide rates among girls rose dramatically, so did alcohol and drug use. In addition, children do not learn as well from home in front of a laptop screen as they do in a classroom with a teacher and their peers.

Lastly, the CDC has to ramp up its surveillance and monitoring. They need to be two steps ahead of where the virus is going. They need to discover any dangerous new variants and devise methods for combating them. The CDC does a good job of following salmonella or listeria outbreaks, so it has the capacity to surveil viral disease too.

PRAYER

Dear Father, we lift our government leaders before you. We recognize the weight of their responsibility in navigating challenges and directing the country in the right direction. Grant them wisdom and discernment as they make critical decisions affecting people's lives. May you guide them in formulating and implementing effective strategies to contain the virus, provide medical care, and distribute vaccines equitably. All this we ask through Christ our Lord. Amen.

REFLECTION

The government's efforts to stop COVID have been a complex and challenging journey. They have succeeded in some areas, and in others, they have failed. However, before we even start being critical about the areas where the government has failed, we need to recognize that the COVID-19 pandemic was new to all of us. There have been many successes in the government's approach to dealing with the pandemic, from swift action and adaptation to supporting the healthcare system. However, the government's role in implementing lockdowns, travel restrictions, and mask mandates was completely disastrous, although some view it as an extension of the biblical principle of putting others' needs before our own. Although sometimes inconvenient, these actions reflect a commitment to safeguarding lives and preventing the spread of illness. In as much as some actions were ill-advised, some were made with the best intentions. Acknowledging the complexities they faced and the dedication shown by leaders, healthcare workers, and essential personnel is necessary.

ADDRESSING FENTANYL OVERDOSES AND OPIOID ABUSE

Fentanyl and other opioid overdoses continue to show up in the local and national news daily. These drugs are the cause of the current drug abuse crisis in the United States. The National Center for Health Statistics warns that opioids like fentanyl are the top cause of death related to drug overdose. And the number of these deaths has quadrupled in the past ten years.

In 2022, the death toll linked to opioids surged to 100,105—over ten times the number of United States military service members lost in the post-9/11 wars in Afghanistan and Iraq. That means opioids are a top cause of death.

Fentanyl is a potent synthetic opioid that is about one hundred times more potent than morphine and fifty times stronger compared to heroin. Just two milligrams of fentanyl is equivalent to ten to fifteen gains of table salt and is considered a lethal dosage. Illegally produced fentanyl is often found in counterfeit pills and narcotics like cocaine. That means some people may not know they are ingesting this drug. This can lead to accidental poisoning and death.

A HAUNTING EXPERIENCE

During my recent presentation at the esteemed White House Opioid Summit, I stood before a sea of attentive faces, sharing a harrowing experience I encountered while working at the Washington Regional Medical Center in Fayetteville—resuscitating an unconscious teenager. As I recounted the chilling details, the weight of that experience hung heavy in the air. The memory took me back to a desperate moment in the hospital, where every beat of the heart seemed to echo the urgency of the situation. A young boy's life hung in the balance as we fought valiantly to pull him back from the grip of opioids. The air was thick with tension, and every second felt like an eternity. Despite our collective best efforts, a somber reality unfolded before us. The room, once filled with the hum of medical machinery, fell into a heart-wrenching silence. We could not save him. The hollowness of defeat settled over us, leaving an indelible mark on my soul. The sign of his parents' grief, their pain so raw and palpable, is etched into my memory. The pain that emanated from them was a visceral testament to the ravages of addiction. His parents, filled with anguish, stood in the wake of a tragedy no words could encapsulate. A chair was thrown in the air in sheer desperation; it hit my leg, but the physical pain paled in significance to the searing heartache of losing a young life to the merciless clutches of drugs and addiction.

My experience as a doctor allows me to help patients who overdose on fentanyl and other opioids. However, this isn't enough. We need to implement measures that prevent access to fentanyl and other substances that are abused widely.

Criminal drug networks often mass-produce fake pills and falsely market them as legitimate prescription drugs. They also use sophisticated ways to sell those drugs to people. These criminals must be dealt with, particularly dealers who sell substances to individuals resulting in fatal overdoses, and should face severe legal consequences.

The federal government must regulate social media networks. Some stories and posts on these networks are often accompanied by code words or emojis that may be used to market and sell fentanyl or Percocet or Xanax on social media. These emojis and code words are designed to evade detection by police and authorities. Platforms like Snapchat and Instagram need stricter regulations to prevent drug-related activities.

International cooperation can help fight drug trafficking. For instance, China has been identified as a significant source of the ingredients used to produce fentanyl in Mexico. The availability of fentanyl, sometimes disguised by drug cartels as prescription opioids (like OxyContin), has further fueled the drug crisis.

In 2022, the Drug Enforcement Administration (DEA) seized over fifty million fentanyl-laced prescription pills (fake ones)[2]. More than 50 percent of these pills contained lethal amounts of fentanyl. Strengthening our border control can prevent the influx of fentanyl, meth, cocaine, and other drugs into the United States.

Additionally, parents and teachers should also teach children about drug use and its effects. Tell your child these risks of drug abuse. Have a calm and direct conversation about this issue. Repeat the conversation often.

Similarly, schools should increase awareness about drugs and create a safe environment for children. They should educate the children and teenagers on the dangers of drugs.

Enhanced rehabilitation access can help. The government should provide greater access to rehabilitation and detox facilities, coupled with the distribution of life-saving medications like Narcan, to address overdoses both intentional and unintentional. I had a seventy-four-year-old post-op hip replacement patient brought in. A car pulled up, and he was dragged out of the car by his wife and son. He was showing signs of dangerously low levels of consciousness and lacked alertness. I gave him some Narcan, a medicine used to reverse an opioid overdose, but nothing hap-

---

2 U.S. Drug Enforcement Administration. "Drug Enforcement Administration Announces the Seizure of Over 379 Million Deadly Doses of Fentanyl in 2022." DEA, December 20, 2022. https://www.dea.gov/press-releases/2022/12/20/drug-enforcement-administration-announces-seizure-over-379-million-deadly.

pened. While preparing to intubate him, I gave him another dose of Narcan, which perked him up. Thank God it worked! I didn't expect a senior citizen to come in with a drug overdose. Turns out he accidentally took too much of his painkiller prescribed to him for his hip replacement.

INSPIRING OUR NATION TO OVERCOME THE OPIOID CRISIS

The White House Opioid Summit was a platform where I could share my experiences and suggestions on how to combat drug addiction and overdoses, a problem that has swept across our nation like a deadly wave. I have also led drug take back day with our local police department and taught my patients and my family about drug safety continually, not just once and done. I recalled a time I left my shift at work in NYC and flew to a hospital in Florida to help a friend in need who was held on a seventy-two-hour psychiatric hold for a drug-induced psychosis. They released him to me where I escorted him on a flight to an inpatient rehab for mental and drug problems. I prayed to God, "Don't let him run off or have a psychiatric outburst." I tried to stay as calm as possible. While speaking with him on the plane, I noticed several molars missing. I asked, "What happened to your teeth?" He told me he had the dentist remove them because he thought there were microchips in them and people were following him. The dentist finally realized to stop pulling his teeth because of the hallucinations he was suffering from. The lost schizophrenic glare in his eye as he spoke to me is something I will never forget. My heart cried, and I was saddened. I prayed for God to help heal his mind and his addiction. I got him into a rehab center that only seemed to care about profits. I had to help this patient and his family in need. So I had to pay thousands on my credit card, as insurance was not accepted. This is wrong and must change. We need easy access to rehab, detox treatments, and mental support. This is a fundamental necessity in society and for humanity. Those with addictions sometimes have relapses, and they must continue to fight for sobriety despite setbacks. He may have committed suicide or overdosed had someone not stepped in. Many Americans need someone to step in.

FROM THE SHADOWS TO LIGHT

My experiences as a doctor on the front lines of this crisis have led me to some conclusions about how we can fight back. This isn't just about treating overdoses; it's about preventing them from happening in the first place.

First, we need to hold criminals accountable. Drug dealers who sell these deadly substances, especially to those who subsequently lose their lives, should face the full force of the law. This fight also extends to social media platforms like Snapchat, Facebook, and Instagram, which may be misused for drug trafficking. Predators lure in kids to purchase a pill that is laced with fentanyl, and the child is found unresponsive in their room the next day by their parent.

Secondly, we must address the international aspects of this crisis. For instance, China has been identified as a significant source of the ingredients used to produce fentanyl in Mexico. The availability of fentanyl, sometimes disguised by drug cartels as prescription opioids (like OxyContin), has further fueled the drug crisis. We need a secure southern border.

By securing our southern border, we can stem the tide of these deadly substances entering our country.

But law enforcement actions alone aren't enough. We need to invest in education and prevention. Teachers, parents, and community leaders must play their role in teaching our children about the dangers of drug use. Ephesians 6:4 encourages us to teach our children by how we conduct ourselves. We must be good role models and teach them the dangers of engaging in substance abuse, particularly fentanyl, and other opioids.

Finally, we need to expand access to rehab and detox services. Recovery is possible, as evidenced by countless inspiring stories of individuals who have beaten their addictions. Medications like Narcan, which can reverse an opioid overdose if administered in time, should be readily available.

The path to overcoming this crisis won't be easy, but by taking a comprehensive, multifaceted approach, we can make a difference. Together, we can turn the tide against drug addiction and ensure a brighter, healthier future for all. And yes, it is possible that marijuana could be a gateway to other recreational drugs. My young twenty-one-year-old patient came in after smoking weed. He was coughing profusely and so hard. He came in because he was short of breath. He smoked marijuana the night before, and it caused so much irritation and inflammation to his airways causing him to cough. I listened to his lungs and could not hear good air movement. I ordered a chest X-ray. It showed he had ruptured his lung, and it had collapsed. He was having chest pain and trouble breathing. A needle decompression was needed to reinflate his lung, which was causing his heart to flutter. Getting high got him admitted to the hospital. Marijuana has side effects, is not safe, and should be avoided. Yes, it has some therapeutic benefits like intractable seizure therapy, or cancer-induced anorexia and pain, or severe anxiety but should not be used recreationally, in my opinion. The only thing we should be inhaling is the air we breathe.

INVESTING IN WELLNESS: HOW TO TAKE CHARGE OF YOUR HEALTH

> Health is the greatest gift, contentment the greatest wealth, faithfulness the best relationship.
>
> —Buddha

The pandemic spread suffering across the country, in every state, city, and county. But when the final statistics are tabulated, I suspect they will show that it was the low-income population and the people in marginalized communities that suffered the most. The weight of COVID-19 has disproportionately fallen upon the shoulders of these two groups, whose plight now echoes through the annals of history.

There are reasons for this, most of which are inexcusable and within our grasp for fixing. Some of the reasons have to do with education, which is informing people how the healthcare system can help them and how they can take care of themselves. In this first section, I will discuss how people can work for their health. In the second section, I will share some ideas that will help improve the nation's healthcare system.

YOUR HEALTH, YOUR RESPONSIBILITY: PRACTICAL TIPS FOR A HEALTHIER YOU

Thomas Fuller once observed that "health is not valued till sickness comes." This is the case for so many people who forget that their health is not an expense, it is an investment. To be clear, good health doesn't just magically happen or drop out of the sky on people. It is not going to arrive on a doorstep or in the mail because Congress passed a law. Good health must be a personal responsibility.

The number one advocate for anyone's health has to be you. No one wants you to have good health more than you. You have to take on the role of being your best advocate, your most active observer, and your coach. No one cares if you don't, except maybe your mom or family. We all have individual autonomy over our bodies; each person has control over their own lifestyle choices, including diet, exercise, and habits. Taking responsibility for one's health respects and upholds individual autonomy. As young kids, our parents or guardians play a vital role in making decisions about our health. They make sure we get regular checkups, eat nutritious meals, and get enough exercise. This is because, as children, we rely on them for our well-being. They have the autonomy to make these choices because they are responsible for our care; but sometimes parents may not have access to the most up-to-date health information or make the best choices due to various reasons. As a doctor, I have seen my fair share of well-intentioned but misinformed parents who end up placing their kids in sedentary lifestyles and other poor nutritional habits without knowing any better. However, the dynamic shifts as we grow up and mature; we develop the ability to understand and make choices about our health. We learn about the importance of nutrition, exercise, and hygiene through school, media, and our own experiences. This knowledge empowers us to take charge of our health decisions.

In my years of practicing medicine, one profound truth that has always stood out is that the number one advocate for anyone's health has to be the individual. I vividly remember the case of a middle-aged schoolteacher whose relentless advocacy helped save her life. I met Claire on one of my rotations as a resident; she was one of those patients who left an impression even long after they were gone. Claire had one of the brightest smiles and welcoming spirits I had ever experienced with a patient. Even her complicated medical history did nothing to dampen her spirits; she had a history of diabetes and high blood pressure and had been struggling to manage her condition for four years. Despite seeing so many doctors, she had never really gotten the help that she desperately needed. Most provided temporary solutions through prescription medicine, but what she wanted was to address the root cause of all her issues.

When I sat down to talk to her, I was quite impressed by the sheer determination and how knowledgeable she was about her condition.

"So, I can see from your medical history that you've had quite a bit of struggles with diabetes and high blood pressure, so how are you feeling today?" I asked her as soon as we exchanged pleasantries.

"I am feeling much better than I used to be before. My turning point was when I decided to take more charge of my health. On top of the prescription medicines, I decided to do extensive research on my condition and to make certain changes in my lifestyle to better my condition," Claire replied with a big smile.

"That's great to hear. Can you tell me what changes you've made?" I asked.

"Of course. I started by completely revamping my diet. I've cut out sugary snacks and processed foods, and I've been focusing on fresh fruits and vegetables. I also make sure to control my portion sizes," she said gleefully.

"Well, that's an excellent start, Claire. Both of your medical conditions can easily be managed with a better lifestyle through diet and exercise. So how about physical activity; have you included that in your lifestyle?" I probed further.

"Well, I've incorporated regular exercise into my daily routine. I take a thirty-minute walk every morning before work, and I've joined a local fitness class three times a week. It's made a big difference in how I feel," she said, sounding impressed with herself.

"That's fantastic! Regular exercise can help control your blood pressure and improve your insulin sensitivity. Are you monitoring your blood sugar levels?" I inquired.

"Yes, I do that at home and also whenever I come for these routine checkups. I've also been taking my medications consistently as prescribed."

"Excellent! And with that, have you noticed any changes in your symptoms or how you're feeling overall?" I inquired.

"Honestly, I have had such a terrible time before with both of these conditions, but ever since I took it upon myself to make changes in my lifestyle, I have never been happier. My energy levels are up, and I haven't experienced any major headaches or dizziness like before. I'm also sleeping better, which is a big relief," she replied happily.

"I'm delighted to hear that, Claire. It sounds like you're making remarkable progress in managing your health. Keep up the good work, and if you ever have questions or need further guidance, don't hesitate to reach out," I told her as I wrote down her notes.

As a doctor, I'm impressed when patients take charge of their health; not only does it make getting better faster, but it also makes our work easier. There is only so much doctors can do; the real work lies with the patients themselves. Even in Christianity, we are often told that the Lord helps those who help themselves. Whatever you want in life, you have to seek it. Even when you seek favor from the Lord, you have to ask for it. Matthew 7:7 NIV says, "Ask and it will be given to you; seek and you will find; knock and the door will be opened to you."

Whatever you want in life, be it good health, you must take the first step to get it.

Does this take some self-discipline? Of course. You have to begin somewhere and somehow create a healthy lifestyle. Stop smoking, avoid illicit drugs, and do not overmedicate. Improve a poor diet and break the habit of not exercising enough. Get better sleep, and do your best to reduce those situations that cause you stress. Avoid people who do not help with these objectives or those that suck the life out of you. If you cannot afford a health club, that's okay, and if you don't have access to safe and low-cost or free exercise areas near you, then you can do plenty in your own house or apartment like squats, lunges, push-ups, sit-ups, stretching, and the like. The Bible cautions us against associating with people who compromise our health; 1 Corinthians 5:11 says, "But now I am writing to you that you must not associate with anyone who claims to be a brother or sister but is sexually immoral or greedy, an idolater or slanderer, a drunkard or swindler. Do not even eat with such people."

One of the main problems in achieving better health outcomes for low-income and marginalized groups is the problem of education. People do not know the healthcare benefits that are available to them, or how to access them. Medicaid or Medicare covers a lot of people, but they don't know what to do. Many don't know who their primary care doctor is. Usually, they are assigned to a doctor, but they don't know who their doctor is, or, even if they do know, they don't know how to follow up. They wait until they are very sick and then go to an emergency room or an urgent care facility. Things would be better if they knew they could visit a doctor earlier in their trouble or see a doctor for a regular visit for a checkup or to have preventative screening tests. This is a case of education or having someone to guide and direct them. This is why having a primary care physician (PCP) is vital.

Education has multiple sources, including media, churches, local government, and schools. But don't forget about doctors—we are trusted sources of information. Doctors need to be a special part of the education spectrum, and this is most important when collaborating with patients in marginalized groups. When doctors see Medicaid or Medicare patients whom they think may not understand all the benefits of the care these programs can provide, these doctors need to take time to carefully explain to them what their benefits are and when they should come in for diagnosis, tests, or inoculations. Many people would lead better and healthier lives if only they knew what to do and what to avoid in most instances. Many people have ruined their health because they didn't know any better; the book of Hosea 4:6 says, "My people are destroyed from lack of knowledge."

They also need to explain to their patients that they should have regular preventative tests such as colonoscopies, mammograms, pap smears, and blood work to check for diseases like diabetes and cholesterol levels. They should urge patients who have never had these tests or are overdue for them to make specific appointments for them right away while they are thinking about them—too many people put off making the calls because they are busy or don't like the inconvenience, and as time goes by, they never make the calls and appointments at all. Doctors at every patient visit should urge smokers to take advantage of a quit-smoking plan and explain that smoking causes more deaths than guns, drugs, alcohol, HIV, and car accidents combined. They should point out that most healthcare plans pay for two dental cleanings a year. They should tell patients which preventative tests and procedures are allowed for free or at a discounted cost. They should tell their patients that annual flu shots for the elderly are often usually free and, of course, point out that vaccines like the pneumonia shot can help fight off infection.

In addition, doctors should emphasize the importance of regular dental care, including routine cleanings, to their patients because oral health is strongly linked to heart health, and heart disease is the number one killer in this country for both men and women. Many people are not aware that their dental health and gums can affect their heart. This is because bacteria in your mouth can breed in your gums and then travel through your bloodstream to the heart. Some of these bacteria can inflame heart tissue and even contribute to some cancers. So, neglecting oral or dental health can lead to heart disease. People in low-income and marginalized communities are the ones less likely to know this, so once a patient is in to see a doctor, the doctor has a captive audience and thus a great opportunity to inform patients that they should not neglect their oral and dental health. Medical facilities or offices should have a roster of free resources for those who don't have medical insurance or have high copays and are unable to cover the cost of their medical care.

Even if a healthcare plan does not fully cover oral and dental work, patients should try to have at least one regular dental exam per year. Just to reinforce this vital point about dental health, there are certain surgeries that hospitals will not perform until you have had a dental clearance. For example, in some places, you cannot have hip replacement surgery until you have had a dental exam and cleaning. Surgeons don't want those tooth bacteria along your gum line moving through your bloodstream to the site of your hip implant or bacteria traveling to your heart where the germ can inflame heart tissue or heart valves.

Fully integrating people with low income or people in marginalized groups into the nation's healthcare structure is challenging. For one, if these people are not covered by any plan, or if they have no healthcare insurance, they avoid preventative and therapeutic measures because of the cost—a topic to be taken up in the latter half of this chapter. For another, many patients from low-income or marginalized communities have a difficult time prioritizing their health because they are busy working at jobs and find it difficult to take off a couple of hours to visit a doctor's office, or they are working more than one job, and it's hard to squeeze in enough time for any kind of wellness checkups or diagnostic tests.

I remember this young Mexican woman who cleaned some shops down the street from the hospital. Her name was Maria Garcia, a young lady with a petite frame and who always had a kind word to everyone who passed by. For a week, I noticed whenever I would pass by, I would hear her persistent cough. One time it was so loud that I had to go into the shop to see if she was okay. When I approached her, I noticed immediately that she looked unwell and had a high fever. I asked her why she had not come to the hospital when we were only two blocks away. She informed me that she worked three jobs and often had to take multiple buses to get to her workplace and thus couldn't afford to take time off. On top of that, she didn't want to spend the little savings she had on medical expenses. There was no way I was going to leave her like that; I took her to the hospital, she received the diagnosis, and found out she had a respiratory infection—she was prescribed the necessary medications and even paid for the one-time treatment. This is just one of the stories of many families like the Garcias who struggle to access health care due to their demanding work hours. That's why the government needs to ramp up community healthcare initiatives and encourage many households with a low income who find it difficult to access health care due to their demanding work commitments to reach out if they ever need assistance. Community organizations and mobile clinics play a vital role in bridging this gap, providing essential medical services to those who need it most.

Many adults are unaware that vaccinations are not just for children. There are inoculations for adults. One of the most important is the yearly flu shot. This shot is either free or low-cost. A flu shot in the fall has a good record of helping adults avoid the flu over the winter or have a milder case. Stopping by a drug store or other location that gives flu shots does not take much time, and what time it takes is far less than losing a week of work from coming down with the flu. People need to be reminded that the flu can also be deadly. It can kill twenty thousand to fifty thousand Americans in a year, mainly the elderly or people with comorbidities. Pregnant women and young children are at higher risk along with those who have a weak immune system.

Other than a seasonal flu shot, the CDC recommends adults keep up to date with other vaccines or boosters for tetanus and diphtheria (called a Td shot). These are combined into one injection that should be administered once every ten years. People who, during their teenage years, missed a vaccine that immunizes against whooping cough (also called pertussis) should get a Tdap vaccine, which protects against tetanus, diphtheria, and pertussis all in one shot. Women who are pregnant should get a Tdap shot at twenty-seven to thirty-six weeks. People aged nineteen to twenty-six should get an HPV vaccine, which protects against certain forms of cancer. People aged fifty and over should get a shingles vaccine to protect against shingles, a rash-producing and often painful disease that has been afflicting about 30 percent of the older American population. There are also vaccines to protect against forms of pneumonia. Pregnant women or people with certain medical conditions may need other vaccines to help protect them. The Bible emphasizes the importance of taking proactive measures to avoid harm and make wise decisions in life. Ephesians 5:15–16 NIV says, "Be very careful, then, how you live—not as unwise but as wise, making the most of every opportunity because the days are evil."

I make it a point with every patient visit to determine whether a patient is up to date on screening tests and inoculations. If someone is in and saying, "I am always feeling fatigued," we work on that, but I use the opportunity of the visit to emphasize and encourage them to schedule their colonoscopy, mammogram, or pap smear or prostate screening to catch up on anything else that they may have put off for too long. Remember, early diagnosis of disease can mean better outcomes.

It's a little strange. It's almost like people fall into two types: ones who are very focused on their health needs and exceptionally proactive about every part of their bodies, having all the right tests at the right intervals, having all the vaccines, and so on, but on the other hand, there are those who for any number of reasons neglect medical tests that could help them—in both the long and the short run. We stress the fact that everyone needs to be their own best advocate for their health care, and this is true, but doctors and nurses have to nudge a lot of them along. We do it because we care.

As I've said, much has to do with education and awareness, but patients have to realize that times have changed, and they need to keep up to fit the changes that have been happening in the past decade. The good book reminds us again us to run away from danger when we see it and take refuge: "The prudent see danger and take refuge, but the simple keep going and pay the penalty" (Proverbs 22:3 NIV).

Below are some things people should be aware of when they visit a doctor, especially for the first time, or the first time in a long time, so they won't be surprised or offended by the questions. Being prepared for a doctor's visit not only helps individuals but also the general health of the whole community.

If you have not seen a doctor in a long time, the doctor's office staff is likely to ask if you feel unsafe at home. This is to try to figure out if there is any sort of domestic or elder abuse going on in their life. Everyone needs to work harder to stop exploitation or abuse.

Doctors also will ask questions about family medical history. The point is to try to discover if a parent had such illnesses as cancer or heart disease or a hereditary illness like Huntington's disease. If so, a patient may be more prone than most to the same condition as a parent. Doctors will also want to know personal health histories, such as a history of smoking, drinking, illegal drugs, prescriptions, previous surgeries, inoculations, and the like. The answers to these questions are important because they can point a doctor to choosing the best path for health, the best medications to deal with a particular medical issue, and so on.

This is important because a doctor doesn't just see a patient for one visit; a doctor prefers good medical oversight and treatment for a patient not just in the present but also in the succeeding months and years. I am not here just to take care of you when you are sick but to help keep you healthy. It helps a doctor to know not just a patient's lifelong medical history—surgeries, diseases, medications—but also the parents' and close relatives' medical pasts because a patient's genes have a lot to do with his or her health, inclination to certain medical conditions, and reaction to medications. The more and better information a doctor has, the better the doctor can provide treatment that will result in good health for the patient.

Something that is often overlooked is a patient's mental health. Many doctors say there is too much obesity, stress, hypertension, bad cholesterol, and endangered lungs. Realistically, a lot of people are not going to do anything about these problems unless they feel good about themselves and feel they can make new behavioral decisions to lead them to better health. They have stresses that lead them to want to smoke, drink too much, eat when they should not, consume sugary soft drinks, and eat "comfort food" that makes them feel good for the moment but that over time is unhealthy. They associate with people who don't help them get on a good path to health and who often lead them to unhealthy choices or even do harm to them. They are stuck in a mental trough that is difficult for them to climb out of and that keeps them in bad health. We all need to be involved and encourage people like this to get into a better state of mental health. The act of compassion, caring, and helping others are ways that are much more likely to result in questionably healthy people making decisions that will lead them to better health.

Exercise sounds rough and tough, but one can get started right away with squats, push-ups, running in place, skipping rope, or just walking. You don't have to buy gym equipment or an exercise machine to get your heart rate up or stretch your body. Exercises take time to do the health work they are meant to do—over weeks and months. You have to be patient with yourself. After a few weeks or a few months, you will see progress. By this time, you should also be sleeping better and feeling better. You are your own best health friend, best health coach, and the best beneficiary of your hard work. If you are really out of shape or very much overweight, it's never too late. Your progress may be measured in baby steps. But you can enlist people who have been trained to help you, such as personal trainers, nutritionists, and coaches. They can get you started and tell you what to expect as you go along. The important thing is to get started, listen to the professionals, stay patient, and keep at it.

A good tactic is to think of progress in terms of months and not in weeks or days. You might say to yourself you want to lose five pounds or ten pounds; make that a goal for a month and see how you do. Another tactic is to determine progress in inches rather than pounds, that is, take off two inches from your waist measurement in a month. Or start exercising for ten minutes on the first day but try for twenty minutes by the beginning of the next month. Never be afraid to start small; it is from little that more is given. The Bible highlights the idea that small beginnings, whether in faith, work, or other aspects of life, can lead to significant outcomes when approached with diligence and patience and trust in God's guidance. It is important to start small and have faith in the little things. Zechariah 4:10 NIV reminds us to not despise today because your initial efforts seem small.

The reason to maintain good mental and overall health during any health crisis is because those most likely to die are the ones who are in poor health. This includes old people in nursing homes whose immune systems are weakened to begin with. But it also includes people younger than sixty-five who are diabetic, have heart disease or hypertension, are smokers, or are seriously overweight. If you keep yourself out of these last classes of people, you stand a much greater chance of a milder case of COVID or flu or most diseases if you get them.

Last, I'll mention one more problem that people with low income in marginalized communities face: unhealthy eating. We don't have to look far to discover why people with low income are often the ones who eat unhealthily. It's easier for them to go out and buy five dollars' worth of hamburgers and fries at a fast-food chain than spend a few more dollars to buy healthy foods like fruits and vegetables. Yes, it's cheaper to buy junk food than it is to buy something healthy to eat. For people with low income, money is scarce and so is time, especially for people working more than one job and for parents who have children at home. Not only is processed and fast-order food often cheaper and quicker than buying healthy food, but it does not require cooking time. Over the years and over time, a habit of unhealthy eating adds up. Spending money on bad eating will cost more—both in dollar terms and bad health—than spending more on healthy food now. Eat more from the refrigerator than from your cabinet or pantry. Eat more from what grows on or under the ground than what comes from a package or a box.

PRAYER

Father in heaven, we come to you with grateful hearts for the gift of life and health that you have given us. We seek your guidance and strength in working for our health, recognizing that our well-being is our responsibility. Grant us the wisdom to make informed choices about our health, eat healthy, and take care of our bodies. Give us the courage to seek medical advice whenever needed and the strength to overcome unhealthy addictions, habits, and anything that might threaten our well-being. May we honor and care for our bodies. In Jesus's name, we pray. Amen.

REFLECTION

Our bodies are the Temple of God; this understanding underscores the importance of caring for our physical health. Just as we are stewards of God's creation, we are entrusted with the care of our bodies. Working for one's health is not only a matter of physical well-being but also a reflection of Christian teachings. The Bible teaches us that there is a time for everything: time to work, time to rest, and time to play. Taking care of our health involves knowing when to slow down and take everything in stride. Finding a balance between work and life through our journey is gratitude. Gratitude is a central theme in Christian teachings; being grateful for the gift of life and for the opportunity to work on our health fosters a positive mindset and motivates us to care for our bodies as a form of thanksgiving (1 Thessalonians 5:18). We need to honor the gift of life every day. May how we live life reflect what God wants for us.

REDEFINING HEALTH CARE: FROM TREATMENT TO PREVENTION

The healthcare, or medical, community is composed of doctors, nurses, hospital staff, public health officers, medical schools, government-supported agencies and laboratories, and foundations addressing health issues. As a group, the healthcare community has the responsibility of attempting to improve the overall health of the nation's population. It's a huge job and consists of one-on-one consultations, medical prescriptions, public health recommendations, public health laws, health insurance companies, vaccine manufacturers, and educating people about health matters.

The pandemic and economic inflation has put more strain on the healthcare community. It has also revealed stress points and places where the healthcare community could have done better and still can. The surge in COVID cases overwhelmed healthcare systems, leading to shortages of essential resources, and the healthcare workforce further faced unprecedented challenges, including long hours, high infection risks, and emotional stress. Many healthcare facilities struggled to accommodate the influx of patients, and the supply chain of essential medical supplies was disrupted. The pandemic served as a wake-up call to prioritize investments in healthcare resilience and public health infrastructure to better respond to future health crises.

We need to keep our focus on improving the health of hundreds of millions of Americans, and to do that, we need to address the gaps in the healthcare system.

There are some diagnostic tests the healthcare community should attempt to make free or low-cost to everyone. These are a colonoscopy every ten years, a mammogram every year, pap smears, and the like. The more cancer we can discover early, the more lives we will save, and the healthier the whole community will be.

Something else the medical community could do is offer more free or low-cost physical activity programs. The middle class can afford to go to gyms and swimming pools and pay to get good exercise. People with low income cannot afford health clubs, swimming pools, or gyms. Communities could offer more and safer parks, more walking and bike paths, tennis courts, and more free community centers where people with low income can get the kind of exercise that wealthier people have been enjoying for years.

In addition, we need more primary care physicians. We need to train more of them and have more available. Right now, the primary care doctors we do have are usually overbooked and overwhelmed. It takes too long to get an appointment with one. Even when you get an appointment, the primary care physician may be rushed because of too many booked appointments on that day. The medical profession must do better to train, place, and support primary care doctors. The health of the entire nation would improve, and that would be a big win for everyone.

The healthcare community also has to do a better job of training and placing nurses, health counselors, and psychiatrists. As with primary care physicians, there are just too few of them, and the shortage is affecting our country. Appointments are too hard to get, are booked too far into the future for people who are suffering, and make people spend too much time in the waiting room. One result is that patients resort to an ER, which causes overcrowding and increased healthcare costs. It is therefore important to promote the training and placement of healthcare professionals, especially in underserved areas like marginalized communities.

Unfortunately, medicine, and especially medicine related to the coronavirus pandemic, has become politicized. It's everyone's job to take advice from trained medical professionals and not politicians running in the next election. Science is what is going to get you well, not buying into the advice of people who want you to like them and will say almost anything that will elevate them to office. The healthcare community has to be more emphatic about seeing that people get good information and not pseudo-information that helps political groups.

People should be especially cautious of information coming from social media. Much of it is simply exaggerated or not true. Indeed, much of it is simply there to shock, to get attention, or to attract followers to an X (formerly Twitter) account, YouTube channel, Instagram, or TikTok. When it comes to medicine and health, false, misleading, incomplete, or sensational information can be very harmful. It can lead people away from making good health decisions. When it comes to your health, you should only be listening to your doctor or the CDC. The CDC guidelines are usually carefully considered by highly trained professionals, are based on science and trusted statistics, and are in the interest of the greatest number of people. They are not always correct, but they do provide good guidance on many diseases even though there were some hiccups with COVID. They handled Ebola, flu, and measles outbreaks extraordinarily well when they hit New York over the years.

If you or someone you love complains that guidelines are some sort of government conspiracy or that vaccines contain tracker chips or other nonsense, have them talk to their trusted doctor or other health professional. The conspiracy theories are wrong, and they have contributed to the ill health—even deaths—of many people. I can name all the ingredients in a vaccine, and none of them are computer chips or parts of computer chips.

More than one million Americans have died of COVID-19; some have died since the vaccines became available in the spring of 2021. Either they refused to take the vaccine—which may have given them a milder case—and died because their immune systems were not prepared, or they could not take the vaccines on account of being allergic to some of the ingredients, being otherwise in a state of health that precluded a successful or prudent acceptance of the vaccine.

The vaccine is not a cure, and some patients who got very bad cases of COVID had to be hospitalized and while dying said, "I'm sorry I didn't get the vaccine. Give it to me now." But, sadly, it was too late. The vaccine's job is to boost the immune system to fight the virus when the virus enters the body. It takes two to three weeks to be effective in this way. Once the virus has settled into the body and infected so many of the cells, a shot of the vaccine will do no good.

A vaccine injection is a preventative measure, not a cure. Today, the CDC has changed its recommendations on who needs to be vaccinated. I have my own opinion about this.

The healthcare community must press for more preventative medicine. We tend to put too much weight on curing illnesses. It makes more sense to prevent illnesses. I think this lack of emphasis on preventative medicine may have two reasons. One is that we Americans don't like to spend money unnecessarily, and spending money when we are healthy seems unreasonable, especially in times of financial hardship and extreme healthcare cost. So, we—and I mean patients as well as the healthcare community—wait until illness sets in and then spend money trying to get the patient back to health. But remember, do what you can now before a bigger and more costly problem crops up. It saves lots of pain and lots of anguish, and it saves money in the long run.

The other possible cause for improper emphasis on preventative care is that we have come so far in medical technology that we tend to think we have a medical solution for any ailment. Need a new liver? We'll give you a transplant. Need a new lower leg? We have a high-tech flexible prosthetic for that. True, we have made astonishing advances in helping people overcome their medical ailments. But these do not eliminate the pain a person went through suffering the ailment in the first place or the time or the money lost. It would be far better to head off alcoholism that destroys the liver, educate about soft drinks that lead to obesity, or cut back on fatty meats that lead to clogged arteries. The medical community needs to do a better job advocating for preventative medicine. This can be done, as noted in the first section of this chapter, by doctors talking with patients during visits about inoculations, tests, exercise, diet, a healthy lifestyle, and the benefits of whatever healthcare insurance plans the patients have. Education is a huge part of the job.

Catching illnesses early enough, or preventing them altogether, saves patients huge amounts of time, anguish, pain, and money.

Similarly, catching illnesses early saves the healthcare industry billions of dollars. Catching any illnesses early means a healthier America, a more productive America, a wealthier America, and a happier America.

So, we should be doing more screenings, more diagnoses, and more health education. If industry, the medical community, and the government all work together, they can also increase preventative medicine in this country so that the therapeutic part can be less expensive and everyone happier.

People probably don't realize that colon cancers are on the rise. The likely reason is that Americans are eating less fiber, fruit, and vegetables than they should and eating too much processed food. The trend in colon cancers is so concerning that recommendations now are to begin colonoscopies at age forty-five rather than fifty. The healthcare community should continue and increase its broadcast of the importance of colon cancer tests. Again, early detection leads to a better prognosis.

I think that as a society we can raise the level of caring and helping. Have you heard the expression, "Each one reaches one"? We all can do better in this regard. If you know someone who needs better health habits, better food, or a way toward a healthier mental state, then reaching out and helping even that one person will have a ripple effect. And when you start helping one person, you soon learn how to teach others to help one person at a time. Then, after a while, there are more people in the community helping the less fortunate. The whole community is better off, not to mention the helpers who will have a feeling of satisfaction and accomplishment.

The Bible contains numerous teachings and verses that emphasize the importance of helping one another, showing kindness, and demonstrating love and compassion to those in need.

Luke 6:38 NIV says, "Give, and it will be given to you. A good measure, pressed down, shaken together and running over, will be poured into your lap. For with the measure you use, it will be measured to you."

Additionally, Proverbs 3:27–28 NKJV says, "Do not withhold good from those to whom it is due when it is in your power to act. Do not say to your neighbor, 'Come back tomorrow and I'll give it to you'—when you already have it with you."

This Bible verse encourages us to always help those who are in need in our communities whenever we can. Nobody chooses to be poor in this life and neither do they choose the families they are born in. Whenever you find yourself at an advantage, share with others.

Romans 12:13 NIV reminds us, "Share with the Lord's people who are in need. Practice hospitality."

Nearly everyone is familiar with a church, synagogue, mosque, or meeting house. Each of these has a congregation. When someone in the congregation falls ill, or has some hardship, others in the congregation offer help and support. A community is like that, only larger. Everyone lives in a city or a county. You can't know everyone, not like in a congregation, but you can help raise the mental and medical health of the community first by helping one person at a time and then showing others how they can help one person at a time. The ripple effect goes and goes; one good deed starts a hundred good deeds.

The ripple effect is a very beautiful phenomenon that transcends boundaries and spreads goodness far and wide. One small, good deed can start a chain reaction of a series of positive actions and inspire others to follow suit.

Picture a community where a neighbor notices that an elderly couple down the street is struggling to make ends meet or even put food on the table. Due to their fragile state, they are also unable to tend to their garden, and the yard is overgrown with weeds. One of the neighbors takes it upon themselves to go and do some yard work for the couple. He also manages to send them different supplies to help sustain them. When word spreads throughout the neighborhood about this kind gesture, more neighbors begin to become proactive in offering their assistance. Humans are a caring, compassionate, and giving species.

During the pandemic, I and most of the doctors and nurses I knew would often offer house calls to our neighbors for free. Sometimes it would be at the end of a long shift, but you sacrifice whatever little energy you have left to check up on some of your neighbors. We were lucky to witness some of the greatest acts of kindness during the pandemic: organizing food drives, collecting clothing for the less fortunate, and offering tutoring services to local children. The ripple effect creates a culture of compassion and community support. It serves as a reminder of the biblical principle that when we help one another, we inspire a chain of good deeds that can positively affect countless lives. "Whoever is kind to the poor lends to the Lord, and he will reward them for what they have done" (Proverbs 19:17 NIV).

Our nation is made up of many communities. We as individuals, but also as doctors and the healthcare community, can all do more to spread the knowledge of and habits of good health. This should be true of everyone and with a special nod to people who have low income or who live in marginalized communities.

PRAYER

Almighty and everlasting Father, we come before you with hearts filled with concern for the well-being of this nation and your people. The nation has been plagued with a terrible crisis that has brought untold suffering and death among the people. We humbly seek your guidance and wisdom for ideas that will help improve the health of our nation and grant us the wisdom to recognize whenever we are failing in our health. Help us foster a culture of caring for one another and recognizing that our well-being is intertwined. May we always be our brother's keepers and through our good deeds, may we also inspire other people to do better. Amen.

REFLECTION

As Christians, when we start the conversation about ideas that will help improve the nation's healthcare system, we should focus on more than just the hospitals and the medical professionals. We should adopt a comprehensive approach that considers the whole person—mind, body, spirit, and social context—rather than just focusing on specific symptoms or isolated aspects of health. This approach values the well-being of individuals and communities. We cannot beat a pandemic individually; we need everyone to be okay so that the threat can be diminished. When only a few people get better, and some are still struggling, then the danger will still be with us. We are called to show compassion and care for the sick, the vulnerable, and those in need. Ideas for improving a nation's health should prioritize access to healthcare services for all, ensuring that no one is left behind due to financial or social disparities. Building a sense of community and support is integral to Christian values; health initiatives should encourage individuals to come together, helping, encouraging, and loving those in need. Above all, the Christian message emphasizes unity and collaboration among believers. The ideas to improve the nation's health should promote collaboration between healthcare providers, communities, and organizations to work together in improving the health of the nation.

A HEALTHIER TOMORROW: STRATEGIES FOR POST-PANDEMIC WELL-BEING

> He who has health has hope, and he
> who has hope has everything.
>
> —Thomas Carlyle, Scottish
> essayist (1795–1881)

It is understood, but it bears repeating: beginning in March 2020, the coronavirus pandemic disrupted life as we knew it in America. A third to a half of the population became sick, hospitals were strained to breaking, and, as of publication, over a million people in this country are dead because of it. Before we had tests, vaccines, or even fully understood what we were up against, millions more felt frightened because COVID-19, even a mild case, seemed, in some people, to have harmful effects. Vaccines and natural immunity arising from the infected have begun to dampen the pandemic, but these have not eliminated the contagious virus. We may be living with it among us for a long time.

What follows are educational discussions of these groups as well as positive measures to take to keep them healthy.

BEARING THE BRUNT OF POVERTY

Poverty is a huge problem, primarily because it is more pervasive and caustic than people realize. Even in America, poverty is widespread and is the unfortunate condition of millions. The official definition of a life in poverty in the United States is an income below $27,480 for a family of two adults with two children. That's four people living on less than $7,000 per person yearly. For a single person aged less than sixty-five years old, poverty is defined as having an income of less than $14,097, or for over sixty-five, $12,996. That's s barely more than $1,000 a month for housing, food, and anything else.

As of 2022, about 11 percent of Americans—or roughly thirty-seven million people—lived in poverty, according to the definitions above, an increase of more than three million people since the beginning of the pandemic. And that's just for people below the stated income thresholds.

There are millions of people living somewhat above these income levels who can barely get by with the incomes they make. Add the recent historic increase in inflation, and you've got millions of people choosing between gas in their cars or food on the table. Throw a health crisis or disease outbreak into the mix, and people will find themselves making even more challenging decisions. In the best of times, more than a few of my patients expressed their deep concerns over whether they would fill their heart medication prescriptions or buy groceries for the week. That has only worsened since COVID-19.

There is no dignity in poverty; as someone from humble beginnings, I know what it means to lack. Poverty can often strip individuals of their sense of self-worth and human dignity and often comes with discrimination, stigma, and social exclusion. People who have never lacked in their lives can never truly comprehend what it's like to be poor. Sometimes, I hear people make some out-of-touch comments, and I keep quiet because it is hard to understand unless you have lived it. One case of a young single mother tugged the strings of my heart. Her story reflected the harsh realities many faced during the pandemic. Amelia was a single mother of two young children: Jayden and Anna. She worked tirelessly to support her two children, but life was still a struggle despite her best efforts. They were barely surviving when the pandemic struck in early 2020, and life took an unexpected turn for the worse.

She was working several menial jobs, but like many other Americans at the time, she lost her job as businesses shut down to curb the virus's spread. Sometimes, when it rains, it pours—to add to her woes, she fell seriously ill. With the help of her neighbors, she was brought to our health center. We found that she had a severe respiratory infection.

We provided her with the best medical care during her stay, and thankfully, she was responding positively to treatment. I must also say, her faith in God largely contributed to her quick recovery. Every day during my morning and evening rotations, I would find her head bowed in prayer. Though torn and tattered, her Bible was also never too far from her. She was making remarkable progress. Indeed, the Lord says in Psalm 91:15 NIV, "He will call on me, and I will answer him; I will be with him in trouble; I will deliver him and honor him." The Lord is always ready to listen to our cries, remove our anxiety, and give us peace: "Cast all your anxiety on him because he cares for you" (1 Peter 5:7 NIV).

However, the joy of healing was quickly overshadowed by the mounting medical bills; the cost of treatment, medication, and a lengthy hospital stay quickly spiraled out of control. Amelia found herself faced with the daunting reality of crushing medical debt. At this point, she tried reaching out to social services and local charities, but the demand for assistance was overwhelming, and resources were limited. Her friends and family, who were also struggling, could offer little help, given they were caring for her two children during her stay in the hospital. Her story was just one of many in the hospital; it highlighted the urgent need for healthcare reform and stronger social safety nets. Fortunately for her, a compassionate hospital social worker connected Amelia with a nonprofit organization that helped negotiate her medical bills and provided some financial assistance. Few in the hospital get this lucky.

Many problems are associated with an income that barely provides housing, heat in the winter, electricity, and food. Americans need access to quality health care, healthful food within a short distance of their residence or job, and to live in a safe building or neighborhood that allows good health to flourish. Many of us take these for granted, but millions of Americans struggle with these issues daily.

Efforts to address poverty often go beyond providing material assistance; they aim to restore a sense of dignity to individuals and families experiencing hardship. This involves meeting their immediate needs and creating opportunities for economic empowerment, education, and social inclusion. Most people are not looking for handouts but a means to meet their needs. The goal is to enable people to regain their sense of self-worth and participate fully in society, recognizing that dignity is a fundamental human right that should be preserved regardless of one's economic circumstances. After all, in the eyes of the Lord, we are all equal, and we should be treated with respect and dignity, regardless of social or economic distinctions: "There is neither Jew nor Gentile, neither slave nor free, nor is there male and female, for you are all one in Christ Jesus" (Galatians 3:28 NIV).

Let's look at just one of the problems: interaction with health professionals to maintain a healthy quality of life. People living below or near the poverty line are eligible for Medicaid, but Medicaid is not a magic wand for sufficient health care. In the twelve states that rejected Medicaid expansion under the Affordable Care Act, 14 percent of adult residents have no health insurance (from a 2016 survey). Even in the states that did accept Medicaid expansion, the uninsured rate for adults averaged 7 percent. Eligibility requirements vary state by state, and in some states, adults far below the established poverty line still need to be eligible for the program. One estimate is that more than six million Americans are not poor enough to qualify for their state's Medicaid standards but not well-off enough to purchase health insurance on their own. That is a horrible predicament to find oneself in—earning too much money to qualify for Medicaid but not enough money to make purchasing health insurance a realistic option.

One of the nurse aides whom I had gotten quite acquainted with at the hospital was telling me one time about her frustration with health insurance. She was a responsible and hard-working young lady; as the only caregiver to her sick mother at home, she worked diligently and made a modest income that put a roof over their heads and food on the table. However, her predicament arose when it came to health care; apparently, she earned too much to qualify for Medicaid, yet her income was far from enough to afford private health insurance. With a sickly mother at home, it was a disheartening game of catch-22 that left her in a constant state of worry. It highlights the absurdity and frustration of bureaucratic or illogical systems that make it difficult or impossible to achieve a desired outcome. In other words, you are doomed if you do and doomed if you don't. It forces people to choose between their financial responsibility and their family's well-being.

There are other problems as well. Some adults who qualify for their state's Medicaid program *do not know* they are eligible, or if they do know, they have trouble getting into the program.

Requirements can be confusing to understand and follow correctly. Even people in the program who understand their benefits have difficulty traveling to where they need to go, sometimes because they are barely mobile or because transportation is unaffordable. And Medicaid service is not without costs; eligible recipients may have to pay for tests, visits, or treatments. In addition, there can be deductibles, which are charges people have to pay for their first visits of the year, making them reluctant to book visits in the first place and leaving them right where they started—with potential medical conditions that remain untreated until the only option is to go to the emergency room.

Disease continues to vex the low-income community in particular because those with low income are not likely to visit medical personnel regularly or when symptoms first appear, nor are they likely to follow a general practitioner's recommendation to see a specialist or to keep up with medications. They are less likely to have the tests they need or even visit the dentist—which might not be covered by Medicaid and can be costly— an important part of good health. It's easy to forget that regular dental checkups are essential to our heart health, and it's one of the first medical services people cast aside when trying to save money, yet it is a critical component of health.

Infections and inflammation in the mouth can lead to inflammation in other parts of the body, including the arteries, which may contribute to developing heart disease. Research suggests that there is a link between gum diseases and cardiovascular diseases. Additionally, poor gum health can lead to respiratory infections; bacteria from oral infections can be aspirated into the lungs, potentially leading to respiratory infections such as pneumonia. Other diseases and complications linked to dental problems include diabetes, dementia, osteoporosis, pregnancy complications, and chronic inflammation. The next time you want to disregard dental checkups, you might want to rethink your decision. Maintaining good oral hygiene, seeking regular dental checkups, and promptly addressing dental problems can reduce the risk of these potential health complications and promote overall well-being.

Once again, many reasons exist why people fail to follow up with specialists and dentists. People might have difficulty taking time off from work or don't want to take off from work on account of needing the hourly income, or they can't find someone to take care of the children, or they find the co-pays too expensive, or fear that one visit to a specialist will lead to more visits, which will demand even more time and more money. But avoiding specialists in this way will lead to bad health outcomes in the long run.

Not eating properly leads to problems that make these people more likely to contract infection or develop disease: weakened immune systems, obesity, diabetes, poor dental health, and so forth.

To eat well for good health, the following is hardly revolutionary advice, and I may sound like a broken record, but I will repeat it anyway: choose fresh fruits, fresh vegetables, whole grains, and low-fat or fat-free dairy products. For protein, choose seafood, lean meats, beans, soy products, nuts, and seeds. Avoid processed food with added sugars and sodium or salt and foods with saturated fats, trans fats, and cholesterol. Highly processed foods are frozen pizzas, fast foods, hot dogs, potato chips, deli meats, white bread, white rice, and cookies. Sugary drinks should also be avoided. None of what I'm sharing here is new. But if more of us ate better, even 60 percent or 70 percent of the time, fewer of us would be plagued with chronic health issues, and we would be in better positions to withstand sudden illness.

Like avoiding making time to see a dentist or a primary care physician, Americans are experts at finding reasons to shun a healthy diet. Even when the spirit is willing, obstacles can be considerable: eating properly often takes more time and money than eating cheap, already-prepared food, and eating healthful food usually requires the time and trouble of cooking, followed by cleaning dishes, pots, and pans. In many neighborhoods, nutritious foods are often not found within reasonable traveling distance, and people need to be more educated about healthy eating. Too many Americans live in what are called "food deserts," neighborhoods where residents have to travel burdensome distances to find fresh fruits and vegetables, lean meats, and so on. Moreover, they might have any number of fast-food franchise locations nearby, tempting them with quick, low-cost meals that, unfortunately, offer short-term satisfaction over long-term health.

But, with some planning, people *can* make better choices, like buying foods with a long shelf life, such as potatoes, root vegetables, carrots, beets, and sweet potatoes. Frozen foods can be stored for long periods in a freezer and often have the same nutritional value as their fresh equivalents. Frozen fruits and vegetables generally are more healthy than canned ones. Another option is to choose fruits that last a long time, such as apples and oranges, and intersperse these with the ones lasting less long, such as grapes and blueberries when available. Choosing fresh green vegetables (spinach, broccoli, collard greens) when possible is best, but frozen green vegetables are just as good and last longer. A good idea is to stock up on staples such as brown rice, dried beans, and lentils. Dried beans have a long shelf life and can be turned into healthy meals quickly and inexpensively. A good tactic is buying from community gardens; more of these are cropping up in urban areas, often in poor neighborhoods where decrepit houses have been torn down leaving empty lots that have been reconstituted with good soil.

Food banks are also excellent sources of healthy food and shouldn't be considered a "last resort." Many food banks nationwide reported record visits by new and returning patrons. The need is great and, sadly, will remain so for the foreseeable future.

One's living environment can contribute to weakened health and thus more susceptibility to illness. Many Americans with low income live in neighborhoods where air pollution can be a problem. In many neighborhoods, despite remediation efforts, some buildings are so old that they may still have lead paint in them and lead in the pipes that deliver drinking water. Both contribute to unsafe lead levels in both children and adults, but the most affected are children, whose nervous systems at a young age can be damaged for a lifetime.

Buildings may also have infestations of vermin such as mice, rats, and roaches, all of which carry diseases that can be transmitted to humans. These buildings are also less likely to have air conditioning to combat the summer heat or adequate heating systems to combat winter cold. Noise can also be a problem, not only annoying during the day but preventing adequate sleep at night. These are demoralizing conditions that contribute both to a higher risk of ill health but also to stress and mental anxieties if not mental disease. And, most upsetting, many of these buildings are "maintained" by local governments.

In addition, people with low income often work at "essential jobs," such as garbage pick-up, factory assembly lines, delivery services, and assisted-living facilities. These are jobs that cannot be done from home, such as the work of lawyers, accountants, marketers, and even teachers. Consequently, many "essential workers" are exposed to more people (who might have COVID-19) and more exposed to the kinds of people more likely to have COVID-19, such as hospital patients and residents in assisted-living facilities. These "essential workers" are also less likely to stay home if they are sick—because they cannot risk being fired because they don't get paid sick leave, and because they need to work—no work, no paycheck. No paycheck, no food, no gas, no medicine.

One of the nurses with whom I once worked suffered from frequent headaches. She was a thirty-four-year-old single mother of two. I discovered that she was vomiting in the bathroom. When I asked her if she needed help, she shared with me her battle with migraines, but she could not take off from work because her health insurance did not kick in for thirty days. I had her rest in one of the exam rooms and bought her medicine to relieve her symptoms. She was a survivor, but she had to struggle through those thirty days.

There are also the problems of high blood pressure, diabetes, and high cholesterol. These infirmities tend to appear at higher rates among people with low income for a variety of reasons: stress, anxiety, and poor environment, of course, but also because people with low income run out of medicine and cannot afford to renew, because it's too difficult to make a new appointment with a doctor, or they've lost their doctor.

Another problem is that many low wage earners are afraid of doctors, don't trust them, or don't quite understand them. They may think that, during a visit, their doctor will discover drug use, unverified citizenship, or a serious condition, or demand uncomfortable tests. They might fear doctors will scold them for smoking, being obese, poor eating, or other habits. Others fear they may catch something while sitting in the waiting room.

So, it's no big surprise that they want to avoid doctors and doctors' offices. I have worked in all sorts of neighborhoods from Harlem to rural towns, including those serving desperately poor and homeless people, and have seen this fear firsthand. I recall working in Corona, New York, a predominately Hispanic neighborhood with many living in poverty. A middle-aged man came into the urgent care center complaining of severe abdominal pain. I was concerned about diverticulitis or appendicitis. He did not speak English, could not afford medical treatment, was disheveled, and was unaware of health care; basically, he was dying. I admitted him to the hospital where he was diagnosed with COVID. It seemed like this poverty-stricken patient had never seen a doctor before. When I'm working with patients such as these, or ones in equally vulnerable groups, I always try to spend a few minutes more than I might otherwise with the hope that they will understand me better, understand the medical terms and the recommendations I have for them. Most of all, I want them to know that, as a health professional, I care for them and want them to be healthy.

Many people with low income living in the United States are at a disadvantage because they may not understand or speak English well enough to make informed health decisions. Accordingly, they may not understand how they can form habits that will promote good health, how to properly use the healthcare system, and how to take measures that can get them better once they become sick. Poverty significantly impacts health, intertwining physical and mental well-being. Limited access to nutritious food, good quality health care, and safe living conditions results in higher rates of chronic illness. On top of that, stress related to financial struggles contributes to mental health problems. Lack of access to health care hinders preventative care, leading to delayed diagnosis and treatment. Poverty creates a cycle of health disparities, amplifying the challenges people face in achieving and maintaining good health.

Unfortunately, as I alluded to at the beginning of this chapter, there is now a new corrosive element underway: inflation. Rising prices make the above situations worse. When people must pay more for rent, transportation, and food, they have less to spend on good food, health insurance, and health visits. Inflation makes bad conditions worse.

Some companies and business owners have taken advantage of the economic situation to double their prices and charge exorbitantly for goods and services. Goods and services that were already challenging for families with a low income to purchase have now become even more difficult. It is not right for business owners to charge more than the market price and make consumers suffer. Even the Bible touches on economic principles and the importance of just and honest dealings in financial matters. These principles can be applied to economic situations, including those related to inflation. "The Lord detests dishonest scales, but accurate weights find favor with him" (Proverbs 11:1 NIV). This verse emphasizes the importance of honesty and fairness in financial transactions.

The same verse is reiterated in Proverbs 20:23 NIV: "The Lord detests differing weights, and dishonest scales do not please him."

These Bible verses underscore the importance of always being just in your dealings. No matter what service you are offering someone, try to be fair. Never let the greed of money cloud your humanity. "For the love of money is a root of all kinds of evil. Some people, eager for money, have wandered from the faith and pierced themselves with many griefs" (1 Timothy 6:10 NIV).

All of the above conditions work to make people who have a low income more susceptible to respiratory viruses.

Remedies do exist. To lower the incidence of disease among people with low income, there should be concerted efforts at all levels of government and community outreach services to:

- Enroll millions of Americans in affordable health insurance programs.

- Lower health insurance premiums, deductibles, and co-pays for people with low income.
- Promote eating for a healthy lifestyle, improve education about healthy eating, and eliminate "food deserts" in neighborhoods and rural areas.
- Make low-income neighborhoods safer by reducing air and noise pollution, exterminating vermin, eliminating lead paint and lead pipes, and making buildings deliver adequate heating and cooling.
- Pay special attention to the people who have "essential jobs" and who are likely to have increased exposure to infected people.
- Increase the number of people who can work as interpreters for people whose first language is not English.

I recommend to my fellow doctors to try, as I do, to spend a little extra time with this group of patients to make sure they understand what you are telling them and that their patients understand the consequences of not following a prescription or not altering a bad lifestyle. I recommend my fellow doctors to ensure, when appropriate, that patients will follow up to see a specialist. Sometimes, that extra minute or two can be all patients need to make the decisions to take care of themselves, to fill their blood pressure medication *and take it.* Something just clicks. Compassionate education works. A little extra time helps people who often feel they are not listened to realize they are cared about, and this realization on their part can convert to some good lifestyle and wellness changes. It's a great feeling to know that your patient realizes you actually care.

I recall an example when a female patient came into the urgent care center having cut her hand while using a knife to open a can; she was hemorrhaging. Her blood pressure was severely high because she had not taken her blood pressure medicine for years nor followed up with any doctor. I stitched her hand and emphasized to her she might have a stroke or a heart attack if she didn't take better care of herself and take her medicine. She cried and told me that if she died, she would leave behind three small children. I gave her a new prescription for her hypertension medicine and referred her to a specialist near where she lived. She sincerely thanked me and said she could live and take care of her kids with her cut, but she couldn't take care of her children if she were dead. She thanked me and told me I had saved her life. As much as it was my duty as a doctor to help save lives, her sincere gratitude reminded me of the verse in the Bible that encourages us to protect those in dire circumstances. Proverbs 24:11–12 highlights the moral responsibility to intervene when lives are at risk:

> Rescue those being led away to death; hold back those staggering toward slaughter. If you say, "But we knew nothing about this," does he who weighs the heart perceive it? Does not he who guards your life know it? Will he not repay everyone according to what they have done?

I think my colleagues would help more of our patients feel at ease if we addressed patients' fears more readily than I think we do now. Some patients simply don't trust doctors. We must work hard to remedy that. I recently saw a patient who was terrified of coming to the office but had worked up the nerve to see me because his condition was not improving—a toe fracture that was infected and wasn't healing properly. With him in the exam room, the patient said irrational things, and to be blunt, was quite mean. I'm accustomed to both kind and mean patients, but this touched a nerve. "I'm here helping you!" I thought. I was ready to bite back, but I caught myself. "Chill out Janette, you've seen this before. This patient is terrified you're going to amputate his leg when he's got a bad fracture that's become infected." I paused and took a breath.

"What kept you from coming in earlier?" I asked him.

"I hate doctors," was his response. "I knew it! You're going to take my toe!" he screamed.

Instead of yelling back, I took a deep breath realizing word choice was critical at this juncture. "No, sir. We don't have to amputate because you're here now—you made the right decision to come here today. We *can* treat your toe, and you *won't* have to lose it."

He looked a little less anguished. But a split second later, he began to cry. It turned out that cancer ran in his family, and he was sure that I would find cancer in his toe. There was zero cancer in his toe, but these deep-seated fears can be counterproductive and prevent people from taking the steps they need to stay healthy.

"For God gave us a spirit not of fear but of power and love and self-control" (2 Timothy 1:7 ESV). This Bible verse tells us the Lord did not create us with fear inside us, so we shouldn't go through life being fearful. He has given us the power of love and self-control, and this is all we need to ensure we stay productive and are bold enough to take the right steps needed to stay healthy.

Another patient, a ninety-year-old woman, came in after she had fallen and was experiencing rib pain along the left side of her body. We did a chest X-ray and a CT scan to check for underlying bleeding. It turned out that *every* rib on the left side of that woman's body was broken. And she had fallen nearly a week before coming to see me! I asked her why she had waited so long.

"I didn't want to be a bother," she responded. "I also live alone, and the thought of making my way over here was frightening. But the pain became overwhelming, and I couldn't stand it any longer." At her age, an untreated fall like that could have killed her.

Another elderly patient was recently diagnosed with COVID-19. She was shocked—shocked—that she tested positive.

"I want to do the test again. I don't believe it," she said. Then she started sobbing uncontrollably. "I've lived like a hermit for two years. I haven't seen my kids or grandkids. No outdoor activity, nothing. I was boosted and vaccinated, and I finally started walking in the park again. I started visiting with my friends again. What if I gave it to them? I'm a horrible person."

She was terrified that she had done something wrong, and COVID was her penance. It wasn't, but she felt tremendous guilt. I let her cry. Two years is a long time to hold back such anxiety—it has to come out sometime; it might as well be at the doctor's office. I put my hand on her shoulder to comfort her.

Oftentimes, when we go through suffering, we tend to think that God has punished us, and we find ourselves asking a lot of questions: Why? Why us? What did we do wrong? Even Job, who was one of God's closest friends in the Bible, went through a lot of suffering—he found himself questioning what he had done to deserve that kind of predicament. "If I have sinned, what have I done to you, you who see everything we do? Why have you made me your target? Have I become a burden to you?" (Job 7:20 NIV). These are the sentiments of Job, who, amid great suffering, questions whether he is being punished by God despite his innocence.

In Psalm 22:1 NIV, even David cries out to the Lord after he feels abandoned in the face of his suffering. "My God, my God, why have you forsaken me? Why are you so far from saving me, so far from my cries of anguish?"

It is normal to question why certain things are happening, but the most important thing is to seek understanding and trust in God's plan, even when faced with adversity and hardship.

I was reminded of these situations when I was filming a segment for Fox News. It was just before New Year's Eve; Pete Hegseth, one of the anchors, asked what advice I had for the New Year.

"Be more patient," I said, "with everyone, and remember to be kind to one another."

"Therefore, as God's chosen people, holy and dearly loved, clothe yourselves with compassion, kindness, humility, gentleness, and patience" (Colossians 3:12 NIV).

PRAYER

Almighty Father, we come before you with every heart lifting to you, the millions of people who are suffering from poverty. All we ask is that you pour your mercy and compassion into all who are struggling to make ends meet, eat, pay for housing, and buy necessities. Provide a way to comfort and provide relief for them through this trying period. And may those who have been blessed with more find it in their hearts to always share with the less fortunate. For this, we pray and believe. Amen.

REFLECTION

The pandemic has exacerbated economic inequality, with the most vulnerable often withstanding the worst of the crisis. The less fortunate in society have been at the end of the stick, and their suffering has only doubled since COVID struck. The experience of poverty and hardship can lead to spiritual growth. It can deepen our dependence on God and help us recognize the transient nature of material possessions. Christians can find solace in the promise of God's presence and provision, even while suffering. Jesus himself is often referred to as a "God of the poor." Throughout his earthly ministry, Jesus consistently reached out to and served those who were marginalized and poor. He associated with tax collectors, prostitutes, people with leprosy, and others who were considered outcasts in society. He displayed extraordinary compassion and performed numerous acts of healing, often on the sick and suffering who were without access to proper health care. Jesus's teachings frequently emphasize the dangers of wealth and the importance of caring for the poor. He warned about the difficulties rich people faced in entering the kingdom of heaven (Mark 10:25 NIV) and praised those who showed kindness to the needy (Matthew 25:31–46 NIV). He went ahead to pronounce blessings upon the poor; He said, "Blessed are the poor in spirit, for theirs is the kingdom of heaven" (Matthew 5:3 NIV) Being poor is not a death sentence; what matters is what you choose to do with what you have been dealt in life. Remember that even in times of suffering and adversity, God can work for good, and His purposes may not always be immediately evident.

GENDERED IMPACT

Women represent their category of vulnerable people. Why? First, women require more surveillance and testing than men do. They need to keep up with mammograms and pap smears as well as colonoscopies and inoculations.

Working women were more adversely affected than men were when the pandemic caused massive layoffs and furloughs. According to an October 2020 Brookings Institution report called

Why Has COVID-19 Been Especially Harmful for Working Women?, in the first three months of the crisis, women's unemployment rate rose more than 12 percent, compared to 10 percent for men[3]. A major cause of the higher jump owed to the fact that women were disproportionately employed in the retail and hospitality sectors, which were particularly hard hit by pandemic lockdowns and consumer fears.

In addition, according to a 2021 Kaiser Family Foundation study, women were more likely than men to go without health care during the pandemic[4]. Women without health insurance received tests at a far lower rate (28 percent) than women using private insurance (45 percent) or Medicaid (41 percent). Additionally, 38 percent of women (compared to 26 percent of men) skipped their regular preventative health visits and tests during the pandemic, and of these, the largest portion were women who had already been in fair or poor health. A significant portion let prescriptions lapse or cut pills in half in hopes of extending the pills' benefit.

More women than men said they could not get appointments with healthcare professionals during the pandemic. But added to this, women very often have stress and depression levels higher than men, and it is well-recognized that stress can lead to ill

---

3 Bateman, Nicole and Ross, Martha. "Why Has COVID-19 Been Especially Harmful for Working Women?" The Brookings Institution, October 2020. https://www.brookings.edu/articles/why-has-covid-19-been-especially-harmful-for-working-women/.

4 Kaiser Family Foundation. "Women's Experiences with Health Care During the COVID-19 Pandemic: Findings from the KFF Women's Health Survey." *Kaiser Family Foundation*, March 22, 2021. https://www.kff.org/womens-health-policy/issue-brief/womens-experiences-with-health-care-during-the-covid-19-pandemic-findings-from-the-kff-womens-health-survey/.

health. Stress can come from caring for children, parenting as a single mother, and caring for children or parents while working one or more low-paying jobs. According to the Brookings report, 41 percent of working women live in households earning no more than twice the federal poverty rate. No matter what the household income, 51 percent of women (compared to 34 percent of men) according to the Kaiser Family Foundation report said that stress and anxiety related to the pandemic affected their mental health, 21 percent in a major way. Add all these together, and you can understand why women's—and most notably young women's—visits to the nation's emergency rooms for mental illness skyrocketed during the pandemic.

One woman I knew from our church group shared how she was losing her mind at home. Fortunately for her, she had not lost her job, but it was hard to transition to working remotely. When at first she thought it would be a blessing to be able to see her family all the time, it turned out to be much more hectic than she thought. The demands of working from home while also taking care of her three children, aged five, seven, and ten, proved overwhelming. She had to juggle online schooling, household chores, and her job, often feeling like she was falling short in every aspect of her life. Trying to balance her job with the demands of motherhood and the feelings of isolation that came with the lockdowns was taking a toll on her. She was exhausted all the time, so much so that she felt like she was losing her mind.

Even the women who were essential workers were finding it very hard to navigate their responsibilities at work and also handle the pressure at home. There was one essential worker who had to be wheeled into the ER after suffering from fatigue and exhaustion. Some of the women had to come from working long shifts only to face more responsibilities at home. Others faced the risk of exposure and the emotional toll of witnessing the pandemic's impact on patients firsthand, and this often led to mental strain. Not to mention, women trapped in domestically abusive homes faced increased incidences of abuse. Lockdowns and social isolation measures exacerbated the risks of gender-based violence. Many women found themselves trapped at home with abusive partners or family members, and this begs for an urgent need for better resources, support systems, and awareness to address this issue.

Unfortunately, there are too few counselors, therapists, and psychiatrists to meet the demand for the help that is needed. Appointments are hard to make, are expensive, and often can only be booked months after an initial call for help, that is, long after the time when help is needed most.

In general, with respect to health care, women are playing catch-up. According to the Kaiser Family Foundation report, only 15 percent of women said they tried to get mental health care, led by Hispanic and Asian women. Uninsured women sought help at a significantly lower rate than women who could use Medicaid or private insurance. Women need to make stronger cases in advocating for themselves and their health despite resistance they may run into from others. Some remedies for women are:

- Get up to date on mammograms, pap smears, colonoscopies, checks for cholesterol and thyroid levels, diabetes, and the like.
- Find out how to receive better care from professional healthcare providers. Seek out affordable health insurance.
- Combat loneliness and isolation. Take breaks away from the children from time to time and socialize with people your age.

- Move from unhealthy lifestyles and unhealthy eating to healthy lifestyles and healthy eating.
- Resist the temptation to put yourself in the background. Step up for your health. You will be more effective in helping members of your family if you are healthy, feeling good, and going about your day with a decent amount of energy.

PRAYER

Heavenly Father, we dedicate to you the women who have been especially vulnerable in times of turmoil. You know the challenges they have faced and are still facing, the burdens they carry, and the strength within them. We pray for the women who have lost their jobs or livelihoods due to the pandemic. We pray for the women who have been on the front lines as healthcare workers, caregivers, and essential staff. We pray for the mothers who have taken on the added responsibilities of homeschooling, childcare, and household duties. Protect them, strengthen them, and bless them for their selflessness and dedication. In Jesus's name, we pray. Amen.

REFLECTION

The plight of women is often overlooked, but the pandemic has starkly illuminated the challenges they face, putting them right up as a vulnerable group. Jesus consistently championed the cause of marginalized groups, including women. His interactions with women in the New Testament, such as the Samaritan woman at the well (John 4) and the woman caught in adultery (John 8), demonstrated his radical inclusion and compassion. Just as Jesus protected and supported women facing social stigmatization and harm, Christians are called to protect and support women who are vulnerable to domestic violence, abuse, or discrimination, especially during times of crisis like the pandemic. The plight of women as a vulnerable group calls for empathy, compassion, and active efforts to promote justice, equality, and empowerment.

MENTAL HEALTH ON THE BRINK

Lastly, I wholeheartedly advocate for training people to become counselors, therapists, psychologists, and psychiatrists. The need is tremendous.

Stress, anxiety, suicide, and crime have all increased. These are diseases not of the body but of the mind. They are very serious problems because they hurt not only the individuals affected but also those around them. These people around the individuals affected by mental challenges are usually members of the family, that is, children, spouses, or close relatives who suffer distress when seeing their loved ones hobbled by mental difficulties, and can even be seriously harmed. The troubles of close relatives might take the form of increased stress and anxiety that can lead to physical ailments such as high blood pressure, ulcers, heart disease, and, some would say, a weakened immune system. Their troubles might also take the form of physical harm in the form of beatings or worse. A study published in *Nature Medicine* on October 3, 2022, is one of many studies that made the connection between COVID and mental illness[5]. Alcoholism, drug use, and drug overdoses have significantly increased since the pandemic began. These, too, have the potential not only to damage the health of the person suffering

---

5 Liu, Shuo, et al. "Long-Term Impact of COVID-19 on Health-Related Quality of Life: A Systematic Review and Meta-Analysis." *Nature Medicine* 28, no. 12 (2022): 2433–2445. https://www.nature.com/articles/s41591-022-02028-2.

these ailments but also to harm—either mentally or physically—family members such as children, spouses, and people who live with those who are afflicted.

As a physician, I have listened to many stories of sadness, and some of tragedy, from patients who experienced horrible abuse at the hands of a family member, neighbor, friend, or teacher. An elderly woman walking home from Sunday mass was suddenly attacked on the sidewalk and beaten with a stick by a homeless man who had a mental illness. A father shot to death his two teenage children because he thought they were possessed. He was mentally ill.

The pandemic has taken a toll on mental health, with many people experiencing increased anxiety, depression, and stress. The isolation measures, loss of income, and uncertainty about the future have led to feelings of hopelessness and desperation. In some cases, this has resulted in tragic consequences such as suicide. Suicide rates have been at an all-time high during the pandemic, highlighting the urgent need for mental health support and resources. Christians can play a vital role in promoting mental wellness by offering emotional support, prayer, and guidance to those who are struggling. The Bible offers comfort to those who are feeling overwhelmed or hopeless. Psalm 34:18 NIV says, "The Lord is close to the brokenhearted and saves those who are crushed in spirit."

This verse reminds us that God is always with us, even in our darkest moments. We can turn to Him for comfort and strength when we feel like we can't go on anymore.

I wish we had as many mental health resources in neighborhoods as we do fast-food restaurants like McDonald's or Starbucks. This lack of mental health resources makes it very hard on people who are not sure whether they are experiencing the onset of serious mental trouble. Because of the time it takes from the day they make an initial phone call for evaluation, three months might go by before they can sit down with a mental health professional. Even when they do secure a consultation with a professional, the appointment can cost a lot of money and may not be covered by health insurance. Over-the-phone consultations may be a help, but these telehealth efforts are just the beginning of what should be sustained assistance.

And if all that weren't enough, mental troubles have long been a taboo subject in America. For decades, nonphysical ailments have been considered a weakness of character and can be fixed merely by getting out of bed early and working hard at a job all day. Other "remedies" have been prayer or living a more moral life. But we now know that most mental dysfunctions do not stem from a lack of character, insufficient prayer, or wayward living. Some have their origins in alcoholism or drug use, but these have roots in personal conflicts or trauma that can be treated by professionals. Many other afflictions are physiological, that is, they have a biological origin. Bipolar conditions, for example, have their source in the way some people's brains are constituted, not in lack of willpower. All too often, mental struggles are glossed over, either by the individuals suffering from them or by relatives who would be embarrassed if their loved ones were revealed to the community to have mental troubles.

Moreover, when media takes up mental health, the reports and discussions are often cloaked in sensationalism: it's a celebrity who harms someone or himself, or someone "out of the blue" goes crazy shooting off guns. The truth is that millions of ordinary people suffer from some mental problem that would never lead to violence but that makes them and their loved ones more susceptible to physical ailments, including COVID-19.

In addition to the increasing evidence of a connection between COVID and mental problems, another study published in the April 6, 2021, issue of the *Lancet* reported that about 30 percent of COVID patients within six months experience some sort of mental illness or neurological problem. Not the least of these are the likes of mental frustration, loneliness, depression, brain fog, anxiety that full recovery will never come, and anger on account of continual fatigue.

What can people do about a rising rate of mental illness episodes in an environment of scarce mental health resources? As a last resort, people suffering from a psychotic episode can go to emergency rooms. Normally, emergency rooms have some staff trained in handling people suffering from psychotic episodes, or they can bring in staff professionals quickly. For less severe attacks, a call to 911 can very often put the sufferer in touch with a trained professional. In addition, many communities offer phone numbers like 988 for people who can take some comfort from over-the-phone counseling. Getting a same-day, face-to-face appointment with a psychiatrist or clinical psychologist is almost unheard of, and many are charging outrageous sums just because they can.

Truth be told, the number one first healthcare provider for sufferers of mental distress is usually not a psychiatrist but a family doctor or emergency room doctor. These are the people on the front line of mental health.

If you or someone you know is in a mental health crisis, remember the following options and remedies:

- Call 911.
- Go to the emergency room.
- Call your doctor for advice and a referral.
- Call 988.

- Call a community's mental health center or public health department.
- Understand that a condition may need long-term therapy and that steady treatment may take years. Find a professional with whom you are comfortable and consider working with that person regularly over an extended period.
- Close relatives and friends can be a tremendous, even necessary, support. These support people need to understand that mental illness rarely is cured quickly or with a prescription. Empathy, loving care, and dedication to a long-term solution are part of the therapy.

Patients aren't the only ones whose mental health was under attack. The number of medical professionals reporting mental distress is sky-high. Nurses felt besieged in the thick of the pandemic when patients overwhelmed hospital resources. Doctors worked on little-to-no sleep.

Stress can feel all-encompassing, even in non-pandemic times. I know of more than a few doctors who committed suicide. A friend of mine was the chief resident at a hospital. He was a fun person, handsome, athletic, and married with kids. During the pandemic, he went to the lake one day and killed himself. I remain stunned by it. I am deeply saddened every time I think about him and his family. The number of colleagues who have died by suicide has struck me hard and made me wonder why people so successful, so seemingly happy, so kind, and so keen on helping others would end their life.

Unfortunately, there are many healthcare givers I know as nurses, therapists, and doctors who are indeed overwhelmed and depressed. Many of these nurses and doctors are dealing on their own with depression or mental illnesses that became worse during the pandemic. They're probably not getting the kind of care that they should. Many are just pushing those feelings and thoughts aside until they can't anymore. I love medicine; I love taking care of people; I love treating, curing, and caring for others. It's a blessing from God, but honestly, the pandemic depletes one of many feelings. There were days during the worst of it when I found it so overwhelming and endless. It was too much for any human being, with no relief in sight and increasing cases of death, homicides, and suicide. There is only so much of one person to go around.

No one is free from feelings of despair or depression. We all have experienced these feelings at one point or another in our lives. For me, my faith, my family, and my mother are my greatest sources of support. I have been surrounded by so many highly functioning addicts, the depressed, and the bipolar, I have come to realize that what's on the outside may not always be what's on the inside.

I am beyond grateful for the strong support system I have and especially for my strong faith. Thank God, I am here. And that you are here. The world is better for our presence, and we can make it a better place if each of us chooses to do some small part—whether that's eating for a healthier life, taking our blood pressure regularly so we don't unnecessarily overburden healthcare facilities, or finding a trusted confidant to share our feelings with. At first glance, doing these things may seem like selfish acts—we're doing them to make *ourselves* feel better—but by taking care of ourselves, we are as well making ourselves more ready to help others in their own time of need.

PRAYER

Dear Lord, we lift to you all those who are struggling with their mental health. We pray that you will surround them with your love and comfort them in their distress. Help them find the support they need, whether it be through friends, family, or professionals trained in mental health care. May they know that they are not alone and that there is always hope for a better tomorrow. In Jesus's name, we pray. Amen.

REFLECTION

The pandemic has brought to light many issues that were previously overlooked or ignored, including the importance of mental healthcare services. Christians need to offer emotional support and guidance to those who may be struggling with their mental health by providing a listening ear or directing them toward professional help if necessary. We must never underestimate the power of prayer either; it is a powerful tool that can bring healing and comfort even in difficult situations like these. We must continue to fight against the stigma surrounding mental illness by raising awareness about its impact on individuals and families alike while also advocating for better access to quality care, especially during times of crisis like this one.

A wise man ought to realize that health
is his most valuable possession.

—Hippocrates (c. 460 BC–c. 377 BC)

Greek physician, *Regimen in Health*
Perfect health, like perfect beauty, is a rare thing; and so, it seems, is perfect disease.
—Peter Mere Latham (1789–1875)
English physician and educator, *General Remarks on the Practice of Medicine*

Although this number will be out of date by the time this book goes to print, as of December 2023, over 647 million people worldwide have suffered from COVID-19, with over 6.9 million deaths. In the United States, more than one hundred million people have suffered the disease, of whom over one million have died—a little more than 1 percent of those infected. That means roughly 98 percent of COVID patients in this country recovered. That is pretty good!

But have they really? Even as much as two years after their last negative test, millions of these patients still complain about infirmities ranging from fatigue and depression to cardiovascular distress. In other words, people may not have recovered fully but instead continue to suffer and experience lingering effects in some parts of their bodies from having had the SARS-CoV-2 virus known as long COVID. According to a study conducted in September 2021, roughly two-thirds of respondents who had received positive COVID-19 test results reported long-term symptoms, even including people who only had mild symptoms when the virus was active in their bodies. Other studies suggested the percentage of long-term sufferers ranges from 25 percent to 50 percent and have identified hundreds of distinct symptoms that linger after the virus is gone.

The distress that post-COVID patients suffer long after they have tested negative does not have an exact name. It has been called long COVID, chronic COVID, long-haulers COVID, post-COVID syndrome, and even post-acute sequelae SARS-CoV-2 infection (PASC). All of these refer to the continuation of symptoms or side effects, not to mention the development of new conditions, after testing negative for the virus. Current research suggests that over 30 percent of people who have COVID-19 will also have long COVID. Patients who were hospitalized are more likely to experience long COVID than others, but generally speaking, we've seen people of all ages and health conditions be struck by long COVID.

The major problem with this virus is that we have not been able to study this problem for very long (it's too new), and we do not have large-scale data on it. Moreover, people suffering from symptoms after COVID-19 not only suffer differing symptoms, but we cannot even be sure that their ailments owe to having suffered the virus. At this time, experts do not know why people suffer from long COVID. But we know long COVID is real because patients began reporting persistent symptoms months after they were diagnosed with COVID. There is no specific test for long COVID, and it can affect anybody at any age.

I expect long COVID is going to be a problem for some patients for a while, but symptoms seem to lessen over time in my patients. As millions of people continue to suffer from COVID-19, the number of recovered patients who will report ailments weeks, months, and years after their recovery might continue to rise. How will we be able to determine if their viral infection caused their present ailments and not something else? And even if we could be certain that their initial infection from the virus led to their current ailments, how are we best going to treat them?

Long COVID symptoms include weakness, inability to achieve former level of athletic ability, insomnia, fatigue, anxiety, body aches, mysterious rashes, loss of taste or smell, loss of libido, shortness of breath, blue toes, chest pains, depression, inability to concentrate, diminished mental acuity (i.e., "brain fog"), blindness, pulmonary embolism, and heart disease. Though daunting, this list is hardly conclusive.

Numerous studies seem to confirm that long COVID can affect nearly every organ system in the human body and the mind. Here's a short rundown of how long COVID can affect various body parts:

- **Neurological system:** Difficulty thinking or concentrating, aka "brain fog," headaches, sleep disruptions, dizziness, pins-and-needles sensations, depression and/or anxiety.
- **Respiratory and cardiac system:** Shortness of breath, cough, chest pain, heart palpitations.
- **Digestive system:** Diarrhea, stomach pain.
- **Other systems:** Irregular menstrual cycle, joint pain, rash.

One of the first such symptoms to gain widespread attention came in March 2020, when Boston-area physicians began noticing a surge of patients with blue, itchy toes. Dubbed "COVID toe," it was presumed that patients experiencing this symptom also suffered from COVID. In fact, a recent study in the journal *Nature* found that most patients with COVID toe didn't actually test positive for the disease. Meanwhile, another study conducted in France suggests that COVID toe may result from a "strong innate immune response" and that people who contracted COVID cleared the virus without developing antibodies that would show up on tests. Long story short: the jury's still out on whether contracting COVID led to people also developing COVID toe, but, thankfully, this symptom eventually resolves after about three weeks.

I've seen patients struggle with long COVID. In one case, a colleague of mine contracted a serious case of COVID-19. He was hospitalized but refused to be intubated and was put on high-flow oxygen but suffered from strokes, a blood clot, and kidney failure. After two years, he is still struggling to get back to normal, still having trouble breathing and thinking. He is seeing a neurologist, a lung doctor, and a kidney doctor. His suffering has been so acute that he told me once he did not know whether surviving the initial trauma of the disease was "fortunate," whether "it was worth having lived."

I comforted him with the words of James 5:13–15 (NIV): "Is anyone among you in trouble? Let them pray. Is anyone happy? Let them sing songs of praise. Is anyone among you sick? Let them call the elders of the church to pray over them and anoint them with oil in the name of the Lord. And the prayer offered in faith will make the sick person well; the Lord will raise them. If they have sinned, they will be forgiven."

In another case, a former US army captain in top physical health who had completed three tours in Middle East combat zones came down with a COVID cough and congestion and still suffered shortness of breath symptoms after eight months. For someone accustomed to pushing her body to the limit, this lingering cough and shortness of breath made her feel like she was living in someone else's body.

In another case, depression overwhelmed a twenty-three-year-old male bodybuilder, musician, and healthy actor who contracted COVID to the point that he did not want to get out of bed, did not want to exercise, and gained a lot of weight. He was unrecognizable. Fortunately, by the grace of God, he recovered and went back to the gym and found the strength to regain control of his health again before he deteriorated.

Everyone who suffered from COVID-19 feels relief, even joy, as the symptoms decline. When the sneezing, coughing, sore throat, and aches subside, patients envision their good health returning. But some of them cannot count on getting back the lives they once had.

Ambiguity

As noted, a significant problem is the lack of data on long COVID. Likely, tens of millions of people suffer from it around the world and in the United States. But COVID-19 has only been around for three years, and long COVID for about two. Much of the medical research community has had its hands full researching, recording, and analyzing the transmission of the disease and the severity of its symptoms once it invades patients' bodies. The medical community has been so overtaxed that it is no wonder they have not assembled definitive data on long COVID. The study of long COVID will have to go on for years and change annually because post-COVID patients as a group will either increasingly return to health or increasingly suffer ailments. Further, the ailments themselves are likely to change.

What to Do about It?

The best defense against long COVID is to be in the best health possible at baseline and of course never to get COVID-19 in the first place—but that is unrealistic. Studies have shown that people who are vaccinated and boosted are 50 percent less likely to suffer long COVID. But because the vaccines are not 100 percent effective, it also means everyone should practice good healthy hygiene, living a healthy lifestyle.

Getting vaccinated, if eligible, may help prevent the most serious complications. Vaccines don't promise 100 percent effectiveness against contracting the virus, but they're helpful. They'll most likely keep you from ending up in a hospital and breathing with the aid of a ventilator. Long COVID symptoms might also be less severe as well.

Further, treatments and therapeutics are available now to help people feel better quicker. I recall an eighty-eight-year-old woman who came to see me recently. She had been vaccinated and boosted but was showing signs of infection. Sure enough, her test came back positive. I called the local hospital and asked if they had any monoclonal antibodies, which they did. (There's bamlanivimab and etesevimab administered together, REGEN-COV, Paxlovid, sotrovimab, remdesivir, and molnupiravir, to name the most common ones, but some are off the market now.) They even had the therapy I wanted her to take! I sent her right over, and they started her on her treatment. She did well. These therapeutics help stop the progression of the disease, and in this woman's case, she was feeling better in days. But those monoclonal antibody therapies are no longer available because they don't work anymore according to the FDA. I also like to ensure all my patients have sufficient vitamin D3 and B12 too.

"But Dr. Janette, don't worry about it! I had COVID once already! I have immunity now!" Yes, that is true. Previous infection will provide some immunity for months, but it isn't a lifetime guarantee. Also, as I mentioned earlier, vaccines provide ancillary benefits besides preventing serious disease—they also seem to prevent the worst of the long COVID symptoms. Today, the vaccine is recommended for the elderly and those with certain medical conditions.

In a June 2021 study of nearly two million COVID patients conducted by FAIR Health, 19 percent of asymptomatic COVID-19 patients were reported to have developed long COVID. Though most patients recover after a few weeks, some continue to exhibit (or develop) new symptoms, which include pain, difficulty breathing, hyperlipidemia, fatigue, and hypertension[6]. Notably, "The odds of death 30 days or more after initial diagnosis with COVID-19 were 46 times higher for patients who were hospitalized with COVID-19 and discharged than patients who had not been hospitalized." I found the results on mental health of particular interest, namely that "of the four mental health conditions evaluated as post-COVID conditions, anxiety was associated with the highest percentage of patients after COVID-19 in all age groups." Depression came in second. Mental health conditions have been on the rise throughout the pandemic, and this large-scale study shows that certain conditions are associated with long COVID.

But how to treat long COVID ailments? Let's take them one by one, though what I have listed as remedies should not be understood as exhaustive.

- **Shortness of breath:** Plenty of fresh air; incentive spirometry, i.e., slow, deep breathing with the aid of measuring devices; inhalers; pulmonary toiletry, i.e., clearing the airways of mucus; and steroids.
- **Depression:** Therapy counseling and selective serotonin reuptake inhibitor (SSRI) medications, which increase the levels of serotonin in the brain.

---

6 Fair Health. "Nineteen Percent of Asymptomatic COVID-19 Patients Develop Long Haul COVID." *Fair Health*, June 15, 2021. https://www.fairhealth.org/press-release/nineteen-percent-of-asymptomatic-covid-19-patients-develop-long-haul-covid.

Children seem to disproportionately suffer significant mental health symptoms. Those with ADD appear to have those symptoms exacerbated due to long COVID. Other children undergo serious personality shifts—sometimes babies become fussier and more irritable, and older children become depressed. Parents and caregivers must keep watch for personality changes because they can signal something serious.

- **Anosmia (loss of sense of taste or smell):** Various stimulations of the senses, time.
- **Decreased libido:** Medications, counseling support.
- **Fatigue:** Proper hydration, natural vitamins and minerals like BC BOOST, sometimes Elavil or another antidepressant like fluvoxamine.
- **Brain fog, lack of concentration:** Exercise, proper levels of vitamin B12, stimulants.
- **Residual effects of stroke:** Long-term therapy.
- **Residual effects of blood clots:** Blood thinners, rarely amputation of limbs.
- **Rash:** Steroids, ointments, sometimes professional care by dermatologists, though some are baffled by rashes that may have been caused by the COVID virus.

One good solution I see is an antiviral medication that helps treat COVID. In all my years practicing medicine, I have never seen a virus that has the potential to attack every single part of the body, from head to toe—hair loss, blurry vision, brain fog, heart inflammation, rashes, and even erectile dysfunction. I took solace in 2 Corinthians 4:16–18 (NIV):

> Therefore we do not lose heart. Though outwardly we are wasting away, yet inwardly we

> are being renewed day by day. For our light
> and momentary troubles are achieving for us
> an eternal glory that far outweighs them all.

I recall a nineteen-year-old professional dancer came into the clinic complaining of a relentless cough. She told me she had COVID about six months earlier. By all outward accounts, this young woman was one of the healthiest people I'd seen come through—here was someone accustomed to pushing her body to do amazing things. She said she had been dry coughing for weeks, and it was impacting her work. She couldn't exercise, which meant she couldn't perform. No jumps, no twists, no pirouettes. She got winded from walking to the clinic from the subway stop! The cough was interfering with her life and her livelihood.

This dancer was missing so much work and so many performances that she risked being let go from her company. She was desperate for help. We made sure she didn't have a blood clot and then gave her an inhaler and steroids to help with her cough and shortness of breath. I set her up to see a lung doctor whom I hope will be able to start her on a treatment course that hopefully will ease her breathing issues.

The big problem we continue to face is that we don't have known treatments that are 100 percent effective. I often tell my patients that even in non-pandemic times, they've got to live as healthily as possible by eating right, staying hydrated, getting enough sleep, and finding time for exercise. These most basic of recommendations, though not foolproof, do help bodies stave off serious illness.

Although rare, children can develop long COVID symptoms too. My eleven-year-old nephew Daniel was hit particularly hard. My family and I were headed to the south of France for a small wedding in the summer of 2021. Daniel had contracted COVID earlier, but his symptoms were mild, and he seemed to be back to being himself and playing sports in no time. He came with us to France and was fine on the plane, but when we landed, he began vomiting. "It must be something he ate," I thought. Only he didn't stop vomiting. Charles de Gaulle Airport was well marked by my nephew's projectile vomiting. Now I was concerned—this looked like more than just bad food. My mother and I gave him some Gatorade so he wouldn't get dehydrated and hurried him into the car waiting for us. My mother was beside herself with worry, but even then, she held onto the hope that everything would work itself out. Romans 8:28 NIV says, "And we know that in all things God works for the good of those who love him, who have been called according to his purpose."

Daniel couldn't keep his head up. He felt weak and could hardly walk. My mother was feeding him electrolytes with a dropper, but by 1:00 a.m., he said he felt like he would die. We hightailed it to the nearest hospital, which happened to be the hospital that treated Princess Diana on the evening of her fatal car crash, and we went to the emergency room. We didn't speak French but learned quickly that this ER was for adults only; they wouldn't see him, and we had to take my nephew to a different children's hospital even though he was lethargic. It was cold; I had to carry him. Due to COVID restrictions, only one person was allowed in the hospital with Daniel. My mother, a registered pediatric nurse, went in with him while I waited in the cold parking lot until one of the techs finally let me stay inside near them three hours later! But until then, the doctor kept coming out to see me in the parking lot because I ended up directing his care. I told the young ER doctor what to do—start with an ultrasound, draw labs, check his appendix, give him IV fluids, nausea meds, ensure he doesn't have appendicitis or infection or an obstruction, and so on. He had viral inflammation in the lymph nodes in his bowels. Thank goodness he improved with supportive treatment. Eventually, the doctors prescribed some medicines, and my task was to navigate the French pharmacies—a whole adventure unto itself. Still, the treatment worked, and my nephew began regaining his strength. I was so worried about him. We could not stop praising God for this miracle of recovery: "I will praise you, LORD, with all my heart; before the 'gods' I will sing your praise" (Psalm 138:1 NIV). Every day I tell him to eat his green veggies.

We spent four days in Paris. Each day brought improvements, but this was something that never happened to him before getting COVID-19. Most kids have no symptoms at all and do well as if it were just a typical cold. It reminds me of a young, healthy five-year-old who succumbed to the flu—unexpected and heartbreaking.

I was seeing some strange long-haul symptoms during the pandemic. One healthy, fit patient developed diabetes after contracting COVID. Was it a result of the virus or the vaccine? In the March 2022 issue of the journal *Nature*, a study of 180,000 people who had used the VA healthcare system found that "people who had had COVID were about 40% more likely to develop diabetes up to a year later than were veterans in the control groups." In other words, thirteen people out of every one thousand of the study participants were diagnosed with (in most cases) type 2 diabetes. The authors of the study caution that these findings might only be relevant for older people already at risk for developing diabetes due to other preexisting risk factors. A question that remains unanswered for the moment is whether metabolic changes due to COVID remain altered for the long term.

My patient who developed diabetes was not an older veteran but a woman in her late forties who was diagnosed with depression after contracting COVID. Her doctors prescribed antidepressants, and in short order, she developed diabetes as well. This is ancillary evidence and does not suggest causation. However, I believe it's possible that the confluence of events in this patient's body could have led to her developing diabetes. Clearly, much more study is needed.

Still on the topic of diabetes, another recent study found that individuals with type 2 diabetes were more likely to experience long COVID symptoms than non-diabetics. The CDC says that those with underlying comorbidities are at higher risk. I've also seen this with some of my patients.

Some long COVID symptoms are so seemingly unrelated to a respiratory virus that you may be wondering if we in the medical community are merely ascribing any strange post-COVID symptom to long COVID. That's a reasonable conjecture; however, after a few years of battling this virus, scientists and researchers have had time to study the virus and study people who suffer these strange symptoms post-illness. They're finding that, first, many of these long COVID symptoms show up while patients are recovering from COVID. Second, when enough people are heading to hospitals complaining of the same ailments, it's time to investigate whether these are related to COVID-19 or merely flukes. Patients with blood clots who've never had a history of blood clots suggest that COVID-19 may lead to blood clots in some people.

The CDC is currently working through several hypotheses concerning the causes of long COVID, such as blood vessel damage, autoimmune effects, and ongoing infections. As of April 2022, there remained no universal clinical case definition for long COVID, but the CDC considers a symptom to be the result of long COVID if it is a health condition that has either returned or newly appeared in patients at least four weeks after being infected with COVID-19.

There's still so much to learn about long COVID, and it's primarily patient driven. To foster a greater understanding of long COVID, the National Institutes of Health created the Researching COVID to Enhance Recovery (RECOVER) Initiative. It's a massive research program whose goal is to solicit patient testimonies about their symptoms and medical history. RECOVER plans on setting up study sites at over two hundred locations across the United States and is looking for patients of every age, race, gender, and other groups to understand the various aftereffects of COVID-19 better. It's a much-needed program, and I believe it will be of tremendous benefit. Learn more or sign up at: https://recoverCovid.org/.

Rapid Reinfection

Unlike the flu, which tends to be seasonal, COVID spreads no matter the weather and continues to evolve quickly. Will we be facing a future where we should anticipate getting sick multiple times a year? I do know some patients had recurrent positive COVID tests despite having been vaccinated. It seems the second time around, being positive for COVID was not as severe, but still, people fear contracting it. Will we ever see a real "back to normal"? Government officials and municipal leaders have lifted public health restrictions—I suppose we'll have to see what happens in the future. But one thing for sure is that we have all learned that there is a new normal, and many things in life may never be the same; we sure did learn a lot from this crisis.

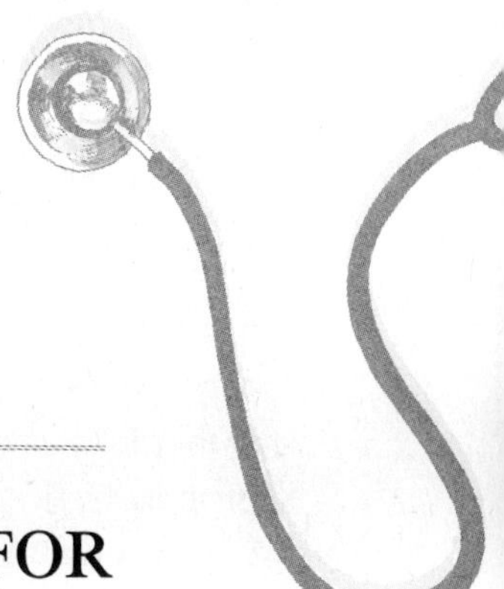

EPILOGUE

PRESCRIPTION FOR THE FUTURE

How many valiant men, how many fair ladies, breakfast with their kinfolk and the same night supped with their ancestors in the next world! The condition of the people was pitiable to behold. They were sickened by the thousands daily and died unattended and without help. Many died in the open street, others dying in their houses, made it known by the stench of their rotting bodies. Consecrated churchyards did not suffice for the burial of the vast multitude of bodies, which were heaped by the hundreds in vast trenches like goods in a ship's hold and covered with a little earth.

—GIOVANNI BOCCACCIO,
The Decameron ca. 1350

Italian poet Giovanni Boccaccio specifically set the series of stories that compose *The Decameron* in the city of Florence in 1348 because that city had been ravaged by the Black Death, losing nearly sixty thousand of its citizens that year. The plague is an essential element of *The Decameron*, reminding its readers that after death and destruction comes rebirth. Boccaccio's characters manage to escape Florence, and their stories, rather than focus on what they lost, imagine a new world and how they will navigate it. No wonder book clubs are rediscovering *The Decameron* as we exit three years of our plague.

Humanity in the modern age has a problem. We are biological constructs. Other biological constructs can kill us—and often do in alarmingly large numbers.

So, humanity has been working to defend itself since the dawn of our species. It's been a tough fight. When you think about it, it's rather surprising we as a species survived at all. We don't have much hair to keep us warm in cold times, the soles of our feet are not much good on rough ground, we can't run faster than many animals that would eat us, we can't digest readily available food such as grasses that nourish many other mammals, and invisible biological constructs such as bacteria and viruses can enter us through cuts, the mouth, or insect bites then attack an organ and kill us that way. What likely kept us going as a species over tens of thousands of years has been the use of our brains.

Indeed, over the last hundred thousand years, the organs of our bodies have not changed much—they are still susceptible to violent accidents, predators, bacteria, and viruses. if we keep surviving, it will be because of the grace of God using our brains to do so. The Lord tells us in Matthew 6:26 (NIV): "Look at the birds of the air; they do not sow or reap or store away in barns, and yet your heavenly Father feeds them. Are you not much more valuable than they?"

HOW CAN INDIVIDUALS AND INSTITUTIONS AFFECT PUBLIC HEALTH INITIATIVES?

About eight billion people share space and precious resources here on Earth. We are smart enough to know when we are threatened, and we are smart enough to come up with ideas for defenses against threats. But we often have fierce debates over which types of defenses would work best, or work at all, or end up doing more harm than good.

Ideas for defenses go by a more common term: public health initiatives. When a threat arises, we want solutions, and we want them *fast*. Normally, these solutions spring from "experts," people who spend their working hours studying threats and solutions. Normally, solutions prescribed require effort and often expense and discomfort on the part of everyone else. That's just the way it is.

As humans, we have lived through several "public health initiatives," some wondrous, some not so good.

For example, when outbreaks of the bubonic plague sickened people in medieval and Renaissance Europe, one response was to send "plague doctors" to affected areas. These "doctors" wore beak-like masks that were a kind of respirator for holding herbs meant to counteract "bad smells" thought to cause the disease. Such "doctors" did little more than confirm and record deaths and very little to comfort the victims, let alone cure them. I would imagine receiving treatment from such otherworldly-looking figures was terrifying.

But another response to plague outbreaks was to move out of cities and into the countryside. Doing so helped both the people who went to the country and the people left behind in the cities because the fleas that spread the bacteria that caused the disease could find fewer people to bite when the populations were not so densely packed.

Bacteria were not detected until the 1670s and, even then, not determined to be the source of disease for another two hundred years, until the 1880s. Even then, the bacteria theory of disease struggled against the long-held "miasma theory of disease," which held that "bad air"—generally, smelly air originating from decaying organic matter—was the source of illness. But rigorous—and sometimes heroic—scientific research showed that not "bad airs," but bacteria were indeed the cause of syphilis, cholera, leprosy, tuberculosis, and bubonic plague. This was a huge advance forward in the quest for maintaining better health, indeed for improving the life of all humanity.

So monumental was the discovery of the bacterial origin of certain diseases that Louis Pasteur, Robert Koch, and other scientists of the nineteenth century believed they were finding the cause of *all* conditions. As a result, they could not understand why they were not seeing the pathogens for smallpox, influenza, colds, measles, and other diseases. The reason was that the source of these diseases was biological fragments ten to one hundred times smaller than bacteria. These were *viruses*, and they were not detected and established as the source of certain conditions until the 1890s. A significant difference between these two disease-causing agents is that bacteria are living organisms. But a virus is an organism that cannot live on its own. It has to enter other cells—in our case, human cells—take over the operations of that cell, and order the reproduction of copies of itself. In that way, it keeps multiplying and infecting other cells, which is what makes a person ill.

Lessons from Smallpox, Yellow Fever, and Polio

Since ancient times, smallpox killed about 30 percent of those it infected, terrorizing people worldwide during periodic outbreaks. About a third of those who survived were often left blind, and others were left with horrific scars. But for centuries, people understood that people who contracted smallpox and survived never contracted it again, even if they were in close contact for long periods with infected people. As far back as five hundred years ago, people practiced a crude form of inoculation in China, India, and the Middle East. They scratched the skin of healthy people, and then into the scratch, they introduced fluid from the skin pustules of infected people. Two out of every hundred people treated with infected puss in this way died, but that was better than thirty out of a hundred for people who were not treated and came down with the disease. Moreover, the people whose skin scratches were treated with infected puss usually suffered only mild cases of smallpox and were back on their feet relatively quickly. Plus, they could count on being immune for life from getting smallpox.

Word of this kind of inoculation spread to Europe early in the 1700s. It was practiced in Britain and then in New England. By the late 1700s, George Washington despaired that as many as 90 percent of the deaths of his soldiers owed not to battle wounds but to disease—smallpox being a chief culprit. Even worse, British soldiers were not suffering in like manner, having gained in Britain better immunity to smallpox and more inoculations. Armed with this information, Washington ordered mandatory inoculations for the American troops. These inoculations were generally successful, and the American army began to hold its ground against the British.

In the 1790s, inoculations were improved when British doctor Edward Jenner noted that milkmaids who contracted cowpox never suffered it again and that cowpox seemed like a milder and far less lethal form of smallpox. Jenner made a vaccine—the word comes from Latin for "cow"—that he scratched into the skin of uninfected people. These people came down with mild cases of cowpox but also developed an immunity against smallpox.

Two similar kinds of viruses cause both cowpox and smallpox. But when a person is exposed to either virus, their body's immune system develops antibodies against both viruses that last a lifetime.

Medicine has come a long way since those early, primitive immunizations, but the path of progress was neither easy nor straight, and sometimes it involved tremendous sacrifice. As noted, people had incorrect ideas about what caused diseases, even when ordering crude inoculations. Only through painstaking and sometimes deadly research, examination, and trial-and-error could doctors and scientists develop means of combating diseases that had afflicted humanity for centuries.

Yellow fever is another disease that has attacked in deadly epidemics since ancient times. Its mortality rate ranged from 20 percent to 50 percent. Frequent outbreaks devastated urban communities. A 1793 outbreak in Philadelphia, then the capital of the United States, killed 10 percent of the population. Napoleon invaded Haiti in 1802 by sending thirty thousand French soldiers. Within months, half of them were dead from yellow fever. The destruction of the French army was so bad that Napoleon despaired of any French empire in the New World and sold the vast North American Louisiana Territory to the United States in 1803.

Eighty years later, an outbreak of yellow fever killed so many of France's finest engineers that the French gave up their attempt to build the Panama Canal and sold their construction rights to the United States. In 1898, when the United States invaded Cuba during the Spanish-American War, for every American death by battle, thirteen soldiers died of yellow fever. Recognizing that completing a canal across Panama would not be possible unless workers could be defended against yellow fever or that Cuba would never be safe from disease, scientists, researchers, and doctors dedicated themselves to finding the cause and a cure. Cuban physician Carlos Finlay suggested that a particular species of mosquito spread the agent of the disease, and a commission led by American army physician Walter Reed was sent to follow up. Dozens of individuals volunteered to sleep with the bedding of sick people, others to be bitten by infected mosquitos. The results confirmed that yellow fever did not spread due to soiled clothing or close contact but rather through mosquito bites and that the culprit was a virus. But the cost was high. Some volunteers who offered to be bitten died because of the virus the mosquitos passed on to them. This was a great sacrifice: "Therefore, I urge you, brothers and sisters, given God's mercy, to offer your bodies as a living sacrifice, holy and pleasing to God—this is your true and proper worship" (Romans 12:1 NIV).

The discovery of the cause of yellow fever led to one of the most dramatic and successful public health initiatives ever conducted. Americans occupying Cuba after the Spanish-American War set a goal of eradicating yellow fever from Havana. They quarantined people sick with yellow fever; they used chemical smoke to kill adult mosquitoes of the appropriate species; they eliminated pools of stagnant water in which female mosquitoes preferred to lay their eggs; and they made all the hospitals mosquito-proof, posting guards at hospital doors to enforce the rules. The authorities also greatly restricted entry into Havana to outsiders. The measures were irritating, but the effect was astonishing. During the decade between 1890 and 1900, Havana suffered about five hundred deaths annually from yellow fever. But in 1901, after the methods of the "public health initiative," the total dropped from an average death toll of five hundred per year to just twelve in 1901, a reduction of 98 percent. By the end of the year, there were no deaths from yellow fever in all of Cuba, and two years later, no cases of it either. Programs to eradicate yellow fever from Rio de Janeiro and Panama also proved effective. By 1940, a vaccine for yellow fever was introduced. This vaccine and the work against the mosquitos have ended yellow fever's days as a terrifying killer.

Public health initiatives *do* work, and the effort to eradicate yellow fever is a sterling example.

In the 1940s and 1950s, one of the greatest dreads of parents of young children was unusual; they dreaded summertime. That's because summertime was when outbreaks of polio among children mainly occurred. Polio was particularly cruel to youngsters; the viral disease could kill them or cripple them for life, some capable of surviving only in an "iron lung," which took over the function of breathing. Americans were particularly familiar with the disease: the United States' thirty-second president, Franklin Roosevelt, as a young man, had been paralyzed with polio from the waist down in 1921. But he beat it and even rose to become the president of the greatest nation in the world. "For our light and momentary troubles are achieving for us an eternal glory that far outweighs them all. So we fix our eyes not on what is seen, but on what is unseen since what is seen is temporary, but what is unseen is eternal" (2 Corinthians 4:17–18 NIV).

In the late 1940s, there was a very concerted effort to find a way to immunize against the polio virus. By 1950, Hilary Koprowski and Jonas Salk developed vaccines based on inactivated polio viruses that could be injected into patients. Salk's vaccine fully immunized more than 99 percent of the people injected. A few years later, Albert Sabin developed a vaccine that could be taken orally. This was shown to be 95 percent effective. These vaccines were highly effective because they both immunized the people who took the vaccines by injection or orally and because they facilitated "herd immunity," meaning that because fewer people carried the polio virus, the general population, including people not vaccinated, was not getting sick. By the early 1960s, parents no longer needed to dread summertime and keep their children away from others. Their children were immunized and could enjoy swimming and other communal activities without fear of this hideous disease. The United States has not seen a case of contracted polio since the 1970s. Worldwide, the effort to suppress polio has reduced incidents of the disease by 99 percent.

We can learn more than a few lessons from these stories of public health initiatives. One is that a massive, consistent, well-funded, and publicly encouraged effort to eradicate a disease is possible and provable. Bubonic plague and polio have been virtually eliminated from advanced countries, and one of the greatest scourges in history—smallpox—no longer exists as a disease in humans. These successes are owed to both individuals and institutions. Individuals were willing to sacrifice for the common good, some to the point of sacrificing their lives. "And do not forget to do good and to share with others, for with such sacrifices God is pleased," (Hebrews 13:16 NIV). Institutions—the Rockefeller Foundation, mainly in the case of polio, and the United States government in the case of yellow fever—were hugely important. So, too, was public support.

Science is complex, and it is costly. Especially when working against disease, researchers struggle against micro-size organic bits that can kill, maim, or severely sicken them. They need expensive equipment and protective gear; they need good salaries for the risks they take and the years of education they have undertaken to fight their battles properly.

Some things could have been done differently in these efforts to conquer disease. The measures against yellow fever in Havana were what I might now call draconian: the city was placed under martial law, and the citizens had to endure inconveniences, orders, displacements, and mosquito-killing fumes. But keep in mind the reward: an astonishing 98 percent reduction in the dreaded yellow fever in just eighteen months.

SCIENCE SKEPTICISM

From the 1880s to the 1980s, science demonstrated astonishing success in identifying the cause of diseases that had terrorized humanity for thousands of years and developed means of preventing those diseases. Some of that science did such astounding work that it wiped out some diseases entirely; they no longer exist as diseases on our planet. Other diseases were reduced to only a small fraction of their former power to cause waves of infections. These successes alone should place science on a pedestal and invoke our awe and eternal gratitude.

But that is not entirely what we have seen. Some of the findings and benefits of scientific research are dismissed or challenged. This skepticism is also not a new phenomenon.

Indeed, there have been "anti-vaxxers" since the time of Edward Jenner and his cowpox vaccine. Despite evidence that the Jenner vaccine was effective against both cowpox and smallpox, some people refused vaccination on any of several grounds: it was "un-Christian" because animal matter was used; the risk of dying from the vaccine was too great; and laws requiring vaccination were a violation of the right to do as one pleased. Of course, to these, counter-arguments were presented, such as the small discomfort to you (both from receiving the vaccine and enduring a mild case of cowpox) is outweighed by the benefit (far less chance of dying or enduring serious illness). Mandatory vaccination laws sprang up, notably for children before they could enter school. Others were passed when epidemics broke out. In 1905, the US Supreme Court ruled that communities could require compulsory vaccines to protect the public from communicable diseases.

Anti-vaccine movements increased in the United States in the 1980s, especially against diphtheria/tetanus/pertussis (DTP) injections, generally required for admission to elementary school. Some people also protested the measles/mumps/rubella (MMR) injections. Science and rigorous testing have shown these vaccines to be safe and highly effective at suppressing disease. Leading to increased vaccine hesitancy has been the proliferation of poorly researched studies purporting to link vaccines to autism and other problems. Unfortunately, the media too often spreads these anti-vaccine stories without proper scrutiny. More rigorous studies have shown that linkages between vaccines and such problems as autism are not validated, but by then, disinformation damage has been done. It is incredibly hard to change people's minds once they've been made up, whether those beliefs in question are based on fact or fiction.

The pandemic has tended to increase the anti-vaccination movement in the United States. Some people believe the vaccines were developed so quickly that adequate testing was not done.

As a doctor, who, like all doctors, studied in medical school for four years and then four more years in residency, we know some things to be true and some not. Medicine, of course, is not geometry with its absolute and undeniable proofs and truths. Exceptions can crop up; one in a million procedures can fail. One in a million men might have a heart attack within forty-eight hours of receiving a vaccine. But there might be no causal relation between the vaccine and the heart attack. Nevertheless, there it is in someone's report: the incidence of a heart attack within forty-eight hours of a vaccine is one in a million. With medicine, you have to deal with data that derives from a great number of incidents and then think about the data deeply. It's true, of course, that everyone is unique and has a unique DNA makeup, but it's equally true that everyone's DNA makeup is about 99 percent identical. This means that a vaccine given to one person is most likely to stimulate the same reaction in millions of others, that abnormal reactions will be rare, and that abnormal reactions may or may not have a cause-and-effect connection that would condemn the vaccine.

All this is to say that the people who have studied the human body for years, who have read thousands of reports, who have seen firsthand the discipline and effort that goes into laboratories and medical research are in a much better position to make medical judgments than someone not trained in medicine but who gets their medical information from media or acquaintances. Even the Bible encourages us to exercise caution and discernment on what we hear: "The simple believe anything, but the prudent give thought to their steps" (Proverbs 14:15 NIV).

Has there been a time when "experts" were wrong? The answer, of course, is yes, if you look back to the "plague doctors" of the Middle Ages or mid-nineteenth century doctors who did not wash their hands between patients. But they did not know that bacteria caused disease, and they had no idea that viruses existed. Today is a different world. We have sterile laboratories that not only can see, record, and manipulate bacteria and viruses but also can map the DNA of their components. We know the chemistry of pathogens and their biological makeup. We also conduct extensive tests and trials that use rigorous logic to rule out false causation. These tests and trials provide an immense amount of data about which medicines work and which medicines don't, as well as the probable percentage of failure and the reasons for failure (people with compromised immune systems or people taking one kind of medicine that would not react well to another medicine, and so on). Doctors are not asking patients to "take it on faith." They are asking patients to accept that physicians rely on reports that have involved years of testing and scrutiny and that a certain medicine or therapeutic should deliver a targeted result with a very high degree of certainty.

It's natural for people to fear or be repelled by what they do not understand or what they cannot see. In the past, people feared "witches," because they could not understand why certain things happened—milk curdling or lightning striking a house. Because they could not understand why certain things were happening, they made up reasons that satisfied them even though the reasons they made up had nothing to do with the real reasons. Milk curdles after a certain amount of time at a certain temperature, and lightning strikes a house on account of ground-to-atmosphere electrical potentials, not because one person has cursed another's house. These are among the reasons why the Bible encourages us to not lean on our understanding: "Trust in the Lord with all your heart and lean not on your understanding; in all your ways submit to him, and he will make your paths straight" (Proverbs 3:5–6 NIV).

Medical science in the twenty-first century is likely not as good as medical science will be in the twenty-second century, but it is remarkably good. It knows how very small bits of organic matter react, and it knows how human bodies with all their organs and antibodies react. And it runs excellent trials and tests. Modern medical science can be trusted. It is composed of honorable people doing honorable work based on scrupulous research. You can count on it.

HOW CAN YOU INTERACT WITH SCIENCE TO HELP YOURSELF?

So what can you do to interact with science to make sound medical decisions for yourself?

First, look at what science has done for you and your families in the past. In recent times, scientists have accomplished amazing feats. They have eradicated diseases that plagued humanity for thousands of years. When you know what they have done and how even today they are improving on the technology, laboratories, instruments, and tests that they used even twenty years ago, you will feel a lot better about trusting what they recommend for your health.

Second, look at the statistics. Almost 250,000 people died of COVID-19 between June 2021 and March 2022—they did not take the vaccine injections that were available for free. During the peak of the omicron variant in the winter of 2022, people who had declined the vaccine were *ten times* more likely to die of COVID-19 than people who had taken at least one injection. Many of these people were elderly with underlying medical conditions. A neighbor I once had was genuinely fearful of the vaccine, she had multiple medical problems, and was not vaccinated due to fear. She caught COVID. She was supposed to get monoclonal antibody treatment but ended up in the hospital. Sadly, she died of COVID. We did not have antivirals at the time. I do miss her very much.

Third, support lawmakers who support science (and not flimsy conspiracy theories), who respect the devastation of health crises, and who are willing to vote for funds to prepare the country for the next outbreak. Support your local public health department and support the measures to combat disease. I often wonder, are we prepared for the next pandemic? I am not too convinced right now.

BEING VACCINATED

It will help you as an individual and by lowering the number of infected in the community. Hepatitis, measles, polio, tetanus, and so on are serious diseases that can be avoided. For example, highly infectious measles can cause blindness, brain inflammation, deafness. Work to elect lawmakers who are not extremists but who respect both individual liberty and science.

HOW CAN WE INTERACT WITH PUBLIC HEALTH INITIATIVES DESPITE MISGIVINGS?

People do not like being told what to do, especially with their bodies. This is probably truer in the United States than in other countries; we like to think of ourselves as rugged individuals who make up their minds and control their destinies. Being told what to do in this country almost always spawns a counter-reaction, naturally. Such a counter-reaction can precede reasons for it, that is, people will take a counter-position first and then second, go in search of reasons to justify that position. These days you can find justification for just about anything, and with social media and the internet, doing so is easier than ever. But be wary—counter-positions can be harmful to your health.

What is really behind misgivings about the government's and majority's reaction to pandemics? I believe there are two general causes: anti-government distrust and disinformation.

ANTI-GOVERNMENT DISTRUST

Anti-government distrust goes back a long way. You might say that anti-government distrust is the founding attitude of this nation—the 1776 rebellion erupted because the colonists did not trust the proclamations of the British king and parliament that they had the colonists' best interests at heart. The Constitution of the United States was written to give the maximum possible freedom to private citizens and limited power to the government. Americans have traditionally granted powers to the government only begrudgingly; they want to maximize their liberties. So part of the resistance movement is simple contrariness. There's no harm in that…until there is. Being contrary for contrariness's sake can be harmful to both individuals and the community.

Be contrary only to the point where you are not running contrary to your health, to the health of those you love, and to the health of your fellow Americans.

DISINFORMATION

"A lie can travel halfway around the world before truth gets its boots on" is an old and alarmingly correct saying. For reasons not well understood, people tend to gravitate to falsehoods rather than truths, to conspiracy theories rather than to explanations that conform to demonstrated facts. Unfortunately, the pandemic has served up a petri dish of mysteries, unknowables, and confusions since the outset: initially, no one was exactly sure where the SARS-CoV-2 virus came from; China covered up information from the beginning; countries have tended to inaccurately report their case numbers and deaths; and two US presidential administrations along with federal agencies and state governments have given contrary information and recommendations. But now we know the truth.

That aura of confusion provided fertile territory for hysterical publicity hounds and social media algorithms to spread a whole spectrum of bad information from whoppers ("vaccines contain microchips that will turn you into government robots") to half-truths. We live in an age of conferences, where unqualified speakers tend to spew huge exaggerations to get attention (not the least of which reason is to be paid for speaking at other conferences). Their speeches, as well as podcasts and proclamations, get picked up on social media and passed along as fact without any sort of accreditation, fact-checking, or counter-arguments. Unfortunately, vast numbers of people can latch onto a falsehood and never let it go. The Bible encourages believers to speak truthfully to one another and avoid falsehoods: "Therefore each of you must put off falsehood and speak truthfully to your neighbor, for we are all members of one body" (Ephesians 4:25 NIV).

The truth about vaccines in general is that they are effective in preventing death and serious illness. Nobody dies of smallpox anymore because vaccines eradicated it. The truth about hand washing is that it kills germs and lowers the chance of you getting sick. It's the number one way to prevent the spread of disease.

So, what is there to do? Can anti-mandaters and anti-vaxxers compromise?

I believe they can. Some of the anti-mandaters and anti-vaxxers hold illogical positions. Let's start with anti-mandaters. Reasonable folks will admit that they trust experts in certain fields. For example, they are likely to admit that when they see a weather forecast on television or the internet, they generally trust the forecast's conclusions. These weather forecasts have been assembled by experts, scientists, and meteorologists who have studied weather for long periods, have sophisticated instruments that ordinary people do not have, rely on weather stations in faraway places reporting on weather patterns, and use computers interpreting huge amounts of weather data. Major media weather forecasts are generally believed to be mainly accurate.

Die-hard individualists might say they can do a better job looking at clouds overhead and holding up a wetted finger to check the wind direction and thereby make better forecasts than professional meteorologists, but they really can't and generally will admit it. This is not the only example of "taking government's word for it" or "taking experts' word for it." People will generally agree that toddlers eating paint in an old house is bad because the paint is likely to contain lead, which can harm the toddler's nervous system for a lifetime. If people believe government weather forecasts and government pronouncements about the harm of lead paint, then why don't they believe the National Institutes of Health and the CDC? People can rightly argue that a weather service is wrong a small percentage of the time, but they should admit that it is right nearly all the time and that health organizations are likely to be right nearly all the time as well; but none are perfect, and when they make an error, it should be addressed and acknowledged—this is what builds trust.

Look at the history of US vaccines and their astonishingly good record of saving hundreds of millions of lives—likely including anti-vaxxers' own and those of their loved ones—while inflicting very little harm. I would ask them to examine the presently available studies and trials conducted most vigorously with many subjects. Such studies and trials end in statistics that show the present-day vaccines are highly effective against dying, hospitalization, and serious cases yet at the same time may cause adverse reactions. Closely examine the evidence, stop believing in delusional disinformation, and honestly consider risks versus benefits of therapeutics for yourself and your community. Make informed choices on your health.

HOW YOU CAN NAVIGATE THE POLITICS SURROUNDING PUBLIC HEALTH AND STAY WELL

The pandemic was difficult, and it has been difficult since the beginning. It presented us with very uncomfortable actions and decisions. People began dying by the tens of thousands, and the rest of us were faced with options for what to do about it. These options were both for individuals and for communities. Decisions by individuals affected the community, and decisions by the community affected individuals. Even the Bible highlights the idea that individual members of the Christian community are interconnected, and the decisions and actions of one can impact the whole community: "If one part suffers, every part suffers with it; if one part is honored, every part rejoices with it" (1 Corinthians 12:26 NIV).

Now, after years of recommendations, mandates, and vaccines, we *can* look forward to a better future. Doctors, researchers, and scientists understand viruses and how they work. They know how to defend against them. COVID-19, like so many other bacterial and viral diseases, has been reduced from a major killer and disrupter of the world economy to a disease that can be generally controlled, like influenza. But everyone has a responsibility in this fight, just as everyone has a stake in this fight. Listen to reason and logic rather than wishful thinking and persons wanting to make political points out of medical problems.

We are all in this together. Keep politics out of science.

Keep your faith strong, and do your part. The Bible reminds us to focus on the present and trust that God will provide for our needs in the future: "Therefore do not worry about tomorrow, for tomorrow will worry about itself. Each day has enough trouble of its own" (Matthew 6:34 NIV).

May God bless you and be with everyone who has survived the pandemic or any illness.

> "I have fought the good fight, I have finished the race, I have kept the faith. Now there is in store for me the crown of righteousness, which the Lord, the righteous Judge, will award to me on that day—and not only to me but also to all who have longed for his appearing" (2 Timothy 4:7–8 NIV).

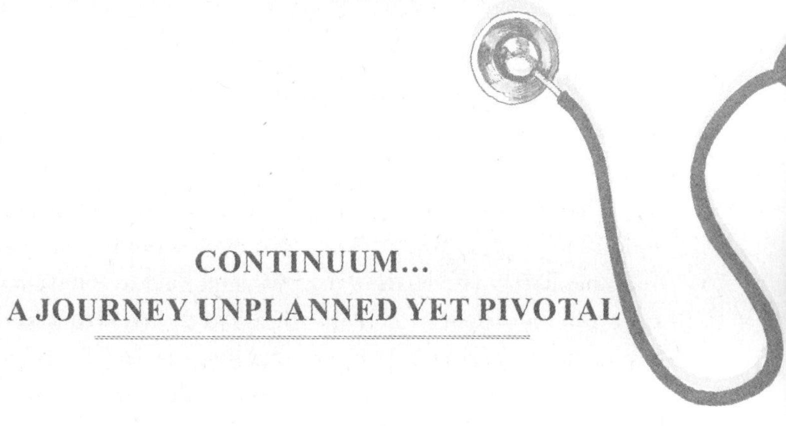

CONTINUUM...
A JOURNEY UNPLANNED YET PIVOTAL

My stories do not end here. At the time of this writing, more and more happens every day. A continuum is defined as a "coherent whole characterized as a collection, sequence, or progression." A progression to what? God's plan. For example, the Morocco earthquake of 2023 and my trip to Morocco were not planned. I was called upon to help, as they were short on medical care after a massive earthquake that killed thousands. Africa was definitely one for the books, and I cannot fail to let you know about it. It has etched itself deeper into my memory than any other for many reasons. This was more memorable to me than my mission to Ukraine. You do not hear me raving about it because it was all roses and sunshine—far from it—this was perhaps the most difficult yet impactful mission I had ever been on.

I went via a volunteer organization called Rescuers Without Borders—the group contains an international network of more than 1,600 medical professionals who are committed to saving lives in areas with the greatest need. Our work was to provide medical assistance, healthcare services, and supplies to underserved communities in Morocco, Northwest Africa. Additionally, we were the emergency response team responding to natural disasters such as earthquakes and providing rescue and relief efforts. Being a part of this noble organization is an honor; I was happy to be of service to others just as the Bible recommends we do. My amazing colleagues, Dr. Hew and Dr. Sylvie, covered my shifts. I am so grateful for them. They are the epitome of teamwork, for without their help, I could not help others. I packed up some medical supplies and headed to JFK airport. The Bible emphasizes the importance of humanitarian and rescue work. We are called to show compassion, help those in need, and provide aid to the less fortunate: "For I was hungry, and you gave me something to eat, I was thirsty and you gave me something to drink, I was a stranger and you invited me in, I needed clothes and you clothed me, I was sick and you looked after me, I was in prison and you came to visit me" (Matthew 25:35–36 NIV).

The Bible further promises great rewards for those who care for the less fortunate: "And if you spend yourselves on behalf of the hungry and satisfy the needs of the oppressed, then your light will rise in the darkness, and your night will become like the noonday" (Isaiah 58:10 NIV). Also, "Whoever is kind to the poor lends to the Lord, and he will reward them for what they have done" (Proverbs 19:17 NIV).

The African sun was unforgiving. Although I grew up in sunny Florida, I could not acclimate fast enough. The air shimmered with a heat that seemed almost tangible, the earth itself radiating waves of scorching warmth. We had to pass through the city of Marrakech where we were met by a whirlwind of vibrant souks, bustling markets, and the aromatic embrace of spices. Marrakech was a beautiful city without a doubt and was even a popular tourist destination. The summer heat, however, can get too intense for non-locals and locals alike. We ventured further, deep into the Atlas Mountains, which were about four hours outside the vibrant city of Marrakech. The majestic mountains with their rugged beauty are now a shadow of their former self after a massive earthquake struck killing thousands and injuring many more.

Climbing the mountains was an uphill battle; I didn't realize I would be climbing mountains in 102-degree Fahrenheit heat. It was so hot; I was drenched in sweat and so thirsty that two or three times I felt I might pass out due to the heat. My experience climbing Mt. Fuji in Japan with my brother Colonel Mike Waltz and sister Captain Julia helped me get up the mountains.

I found the inner resolve to keep moving forward knowing that thousands of families living upon rubble depended on the medical aid we brought. We could hear the cries and mourning of young children and mothers echoing through the rugged terrain. These mountains were home to 2.5 million villagers, isolated from modern conveniences and with little or no access to health care. The community was so remote, that there was no 911 to call for help in case of medical emergencies. This meant that illnesses could often be a death sentence as the villagers lacked the means to afford transportation to distant towns or to pay for medical care. It is reality, a harsh reminder of the stark disparities that exist in our world, and it broke my heart in many ways.

I was reminded of how we often take for granted the privileges that we have in the United States. The Bible addresses the idea of disparities and inequalities in the world; the disparities between the poor and rich existed even in the Bible. But we are always encouraged to act fairly, treat everyone with kindness, and do everything in our power to even the playing field: "Is not this the kind of fasting I have chosen: to lose the chains of injustice and untie the cords of the yoke, to set the oppressed free and break every yoke? Is it not to share your food with the hungry and to provide the poor wanderer with shelter—when you see the naked, to clothe them, and not to turn away from your own flesh and blood?" (Isaiah 58:6–7 NIV).

Here I was, determined to do my part in making the world a better place. My heart sank as I gazed upon the scene that lay ahead of me: crumbled buildings and debris were scattered across the mountain villages, and the once-thriving communities now lie in ruins. The survivors were in a state of shock and desperation, their eyes reflecting the trauma they had endured.

We wasted no time setting up a makeshift triage center where the wounded were brought in, many with injuries that ranged from broken bones to severe trauma and infected wounds. The absence of proper healthcare facilities in this remote region had magnified the suffering, and we were their hope. With limited resources, we had to make every moment count and ensure we took care of as many as we could.

I, along with my fellow doctors and nurses, immediately got to work. The injured were triaged, and we prioritized those in critical condition. The sound of cries and moans filled the air as we did our best to provide comfort and treatment. Amid this chaos, the spirit of teamwork was palpable as we worked together to save lives.

I learned a lesson that even in the mountains of Africa, I needed to triage. I could not see everyone and needed to reserve my energy for those who needed it most. Hundreds flocked toward us because they either never saw a doctor or hadn't seen one in years, but my time and resources needed to be used wisely. I wondered, what if we weren't there—what would have happened? I realized that they would die if not healed naturally. They were suffering from asthma exacerbations, abdominal pain, ulcers, headaches, wounds, infections, and a lot more.

One young girl lay paralyzed with flies swarming around her; I used a bottle cap to pour sips of water into her mouth. One young boy was brought in with a large laceration from knee to ankle after being caught underneath cement rubble. He needed a surgeon, but there were none. I washed out his leg and stapled the wound together and started him on antibiotics. I knew I would move on to the next village, so I taught his father how to remove the staples in two weeks. If not properly cared for, it could result in infection or loss of limb. There were also lots of sick babies vomiting with diarrhea and rashes. It was a blessing we had the medicine and supplies to care for them all. My heart ached for the beautiful, orphaned children; they go to school in tents, and they were living in tents because their homes were destroyed by the earthquake.

"Death has climbed in through our windows and has entered our fortresses; it has removed the children from the streets and the young men from the public squares" (Jeremiah 9:21 NIV).

We went to different villages; there were about two hundred. I had already seen 150 patients and was about to collapse; I was so exhausted, drenched in sweat, and sunburned. I was barely holding myself together, but sometimes I would gaze up and marvel at the majestic mountains. The mountains were so beautiful. I miss it. I miss Morocco. I would rather be there right now than in New York City.

At the last village, there was a brief windstorm of sand. We all paused and shut our eyes tight for about five minutes until it passed (I felt like Indiana Jones in Petra, the temple of doom, don't look). On our way out, a group of villagers surrounding a young teen girl came screaming toward our vehicle with her hand over her eye. I wondered what the heck was going on. She was screaming in pain, "My eye, my eye!" I jumped out of the car and opened her eye with difficulty. I didn't have the equipment for eyes that I have in the US. I found in an old box some saline syringes. I grabbed a handful and started flushing out her eyes. It's all I had. After a few flushes, she continued to be in pain, screaming. I continued to wash, and finally, I saw a dime-size sharp shard of plastic emerge from her eye. I continued to try to flush it out and remove it. It was stuck; I needed to gently remove it without causing internal damage. I had no lidocaine drops to relieve her pain, which I would have killed for during that time. I continued to aggressively flush, and finally, it came out. I wondered if she would have lost her eye or gone blind. Luckily, I found a tiny tube of antibiotic ointment and placed some in her eye to soothe her eye and prevent infection. The blessing to have the basic necessity to take care of her in the middle of the mountains of Africa where there were no eye doctors or ob-gyns or cardiologists—it was just me and my team and God by our side.

I am so happy and content that I can use my gifts to be a blessing to others. The Bible underscores the idea that serving others, especially those in need, is not only a noble and selfless act but also a source of joy, blessings, and an expression of love and faith: "Each of you should use whatever gift you have received to serve others, as faithful stewards of God's grace in its various forms" (1 Peter 4:10 NIV).

We plan to build a small health clinic for them and have it manned by a nurse or doctor. We are still working on it and plan to teach basic life support and wound care on our next trip. The village leader insisted I sit down and make couscous with her for the village; it was a gesture of respect and gratitude. It's a traditional Moroccan dish. I love Morocco, I love the country, beautiful people, and beautiful culture. I pray for their safety and healing. My heart is still there.

I am blessed to have the honor of serving God by caring for others. I don't know what else I would do with my life. I just wish I spoke French like they do. My Arabic wasn't as helpful as I thought it could be. Back in NYC, people get sick or chip a nail, and they go to a doctor or urgent care. We have it so easy in the US. My perspective is renewed. In the meantime, another earthquake, even bigger, struck Afghanistan, there's war in Armenia, and now Israel and Gaza. I pray for peace for all.

As I reflect on a journey that transcends the chaotic hustle of the emergency room or a war-torn, poverty-stricken country, each journey, a testament to the miracles I witnessed and the challenges I faced as a doctor, has brought me closer to Christ and the essence of healing. In the unpredictable symphony of life and death, I have realized the interconnection between medicine and faith. Beyond the tests and prescription pads, there exists a realm where miracles unfold and hope springs eternal. As I bid farewell to the pages of this book, I extend an invitation for you, dear reader, to embrace the miracles within your own life, find solace in faith during life's storms, and extend compassion to those in need.

With humility, love, and abundant faith in our Lord, I look forward to the future miracles I have yet to see.

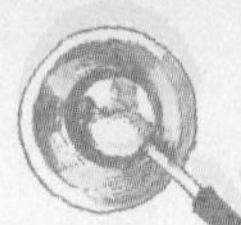

ACKNOWLEDGMENTS

To God, for granting me the strength, wisdom, and grace to overcome challenges and witness the miracles that inspire this book.

To everyone who has walked this journey with me, your support has been invaluable.

To my family, Danny, Christine, Christopher, lil Hayat, JonPaul, Zain, Dina, Jaclyn, Milan, Daniel, Anthony, Brenda, Anderson, Mike, Julia, and Armie, whose boundless love and encouragement have been my foundation and the heartbeat of my existence.

To my friends and colleagues, whose unwavering support and belief in me have fueled my determination and been the lifeline that kept me going, most notably Michelle Drake, Dr. Karen Semones, Dr. Phil Hew, Dr. Sammy Turner, Michelle Geskey, Sean Linnehan, and Dr. Greg Olsen for supporting our medical missions in times of crisis.

Special thanks to my hero and sister, Captain Julia Nesheiwat, and my brother, Colonel Mike Waltz, for your extraordinary contributions and inspiration to me and the country.

To Dana Perino, Ainsley Earhardt, Neil Cavuto, and Kennedy, for your kindness and support.

To all my readers, thank you for embarking on this journey of faith, hope, and healing. Together, we explore the ups and downs of life.

To my lovely sister, Dina, who helped while I was on the front lines taking care of patients.

To Oksana, who assisted me with translations in Ukraine. You're a beacon of light!

To Aleigha Koss for working with me on every aspect of my book—you're amazing; Anthony Ziccardi and Dan Bongino, thank you for giving me the opportunity to share my story. Barbara Richter and Diana Rangraves, for your work and support.

Finally, to my mom, Nurse Hayat, whose hands have healed countless lives and whose beautiful heart has touched even more. Your steadfast compassion, dedication, and strength have been a constant inspiration to us all. You have shown me the true meaning of care and the power of a kind heart. Your love and living a life of servitude and giving have been my guiding light, and your tireless commitment to helping others has illuminated my path and ignited my own passion for medicine. I am blessed to call you Mom.

This book is a testament to the miracles I've witnessed, reflecting the values and dedication you instilled in me. Thank you, mom, for being my first teacher, my role model, my guiding star and my greatest supporter. This journey is as much yours as it is mine.

With all my love and gratitude,
Dr. Janette Nesheiwat